ikioo

21st CENTURY MEDICINE

ARTIFICIAL INTELLIGENCE FOR HEALTH PROFESSIONALS

ikioo ® - 21st Century Medicine:
Artificial Intelligence for Health Professionals
Copyright © 2017 Ayman Salem, MD
Published by BARQUQ

For further information, please contact:
BARQUQ
191 S. Buena Vista Street, Suite # 370
Burbank CA 91505

Printed in the United States of America

Design by
Arbor Services, Inc.
http://www.arborservices.co/

1. Title   2. Author   3. Medical

Library of Congress Control Number: 2017901269

ISBN: 978-0-9975096-1-8

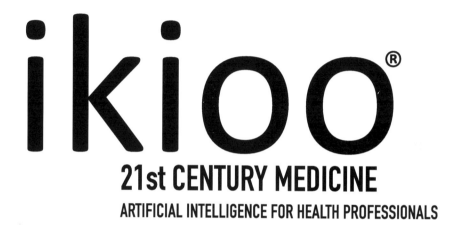

ikioo®

21st CENTURY MEDICINE

ARTIFICIAL INTELLIGENCE FOR HEALTH PROFESSIONALS

By

Dr. Ayman Salem

BARQUQ

Glory and Grace Be to God

To my mother and late father who taught me about medicine at a young age, and who instilled in my heart to selflessly care about all humans. To my wife Meghan and children Altarek and Aya who make life so much worth living. And to sharing the American dream, which against all odds makes the impossible, possible.

Contents

Foreword

Revised Hippocratic Oath 1964
by Dr. Louis Lasagna (February 22, 1923 – August 6, 2003)
an American physician and professor of medicine.

I swear to fulfill, to the best of my ability and judgment, this covenant:

I will respect the hard-won scientific gains of those physicians in whose steps I walk, and gladly share such knowledge as is mine with those who are to follow.

I will apply, for the benefit of the sick, all measures [that] are required, avoiding those twin traps of overtreatment and therapeutic nihilism.

I will remember that there is art to medicine as well as science, and that warmth, sympathy, and understanding may outweigh the surgeon's knife or the chemist's drug.

I will not be ashamed to say, "I know not," nor will I fail to call in my colleagues when the skills of another are needed for a patient's recovery.

I will respect the privacy of my patients, for their problems are not disclosed to me that the world may know. Most especially must I tread with care in matters of life and death. If it is given me to save a life, all thanks. But it may also be within my power to take a life; this awesome responsibility must be faced with great humbleness and awareness of my own frailty. Above all, I must not play at God.

I will remember that I do not treat a fever chart or a cancerous growth, but a sick human being, whose illness may affect the person's family and economic stability. My responsibility includes these related problems, if I am to care adequately for the sick.

I will prevent disease whenever I can, for prevention is preferable to cure.

I will remember that I remain a member of society, with special obligations to all my fellow human beings, those sound of mind and body as well as the infirm.

If I do not violate this oath, may I enjoy life and art, respected while I live and remembered with affection thereafter. May I always act so as to preserve the finest traditions of my calling and may I long experience the joy of healing those who seek my help.

Introduction

At ikioo® Technologies, Inc., we are a group of innovative healthcare providers and software engineers that voluntarily subscribe to the doctrine of British author Sir Arthur Conan Doyle and his "consulting detective" Sherlock Holmes. As most people are familiar, Doyle's stories are narrated by Holmes's friend and liaison, Dr. Watson, who shares in the adventures and investigations. The phrase "Elementary, my dear Watson" is what sets Holmes and Watson apart.

Artificial intelligence and artificial superintelligence is uncharted territory for many of us in healthcare. We see the potential and hear the alarm bells simultaneously. The simple premise of putting all our human health conscience into a machine's deep learning algorithm to be carried elsewhere raises serious concerns. But at the same time, such advances offer tremendous opportunities for advancement and improvement in healthcare.

Intuition and creativity are currently hot topics within the field of artificial intelligence. Google's DeepMind Alphago® clearly demonstrated a glimpse of that vision. I remember during my research days in applied neurosciences for Parkinson's disease, the question of differentiating between the brain and the mind always came up. Embedding virtual anatomic structures like the virtual hippocampus into an actual machine embraces a whole new frontier. And having our collective thoughts and intuitions in healthcare as vectors in a machine can be quite exhilarating.

The term "approach" encompasses what we do in healthcare. However, it is not necessarily a simple problem with a straightforward solution. The third and fourth options on a decision tree list might be more appropriate than the first and second choices. This is where human intuition and judgment come into play, and as a mentor once instructed me, we must temper justice with mercy. While machines do not have that level of capacity and sophistication, I have no doubt that one day machines will reach increasing levels of wisdom that will continually enhance human intelligence.

Humanity as well as healthcare providers will benefit greatly from advances in artificial intelligence in healthcare. In referring back to Doyle's stories, sidekicks tend to have more freedom in misadventures and in making mistakes than the hero. But it is the hero that chooses to take the path less traveled. It was Holmes's eccentric interests and unique perspectives that made him adept in solving many problems, much to the amazement and bewilderment of Watson. For healthcare, artificial intelligence and machine deep learning systems portray such a path.

Machine deep learning systems should naturally follow the same long-standing established traditions of rigorous training for our profession. Preset qualifiers and standards must be established and implemented. Regardless, deep machine learning offers a great opportunity to enhance the practice of medicine. Patients have the potential to benefit from unparalleled efficiencies in seeking medical advice, tracking their health, and fulfilling medical recommendations by their healthcare providers.

Healthcare regulators should appreciate this moment in history and support more innovation and progress in these areas. The landscape in healthcare will undergo major changes as a result, and some healthcare stakeholders, if not most, will resist change. Healthcare consumers will ultimately demand appropriate healthcare reforms via their duly elected representatives, so whether embraced or not, change will come.

This book is an effort to put into simple terms a complex issue from one healthcare provider's viewpoint. It reflects the current state of affairs in US healthcare in the beginnings of the twenty-first century and ushers in the sea of positive changes that lie ahead. It is also an open invitation to share thoughts and ideas for all involved, to better serve those who are most in need.

Ayman Salem, MD

CHAPTER 1

Return to "Nuanced Medicine" for the Twenty-First Century

What Is Nuanced Medicine?

Great advances in medicine occur when subtle distinctions are recognized that subsequently prompt change. For example, at the turn of the twenty-first century, over thirty thousand diseases had been identified with diagnosis and management algorithms available for approximately ten thousand of these diseases. By twentieth-century standards, this reflects quite the advancement. In addition, major scientific breakthroughs in cancer treatment, infectious disease therapies, and genetics have evolved as well. The more nuanced medicine becomes, the better is the care that can be rendered for a variety of health disorders.

In healthcare, professionals are trained with a focus on the acute and chronic care management of disease. In other words, what is labeled as "healthcare" could be more accurately termed "disease care," and healthcare professionals referred to as disease care professionals. As disease care delivery has become increasingly nuanced, the costs associated with this approach have been substantial. Escalating costs of disease care, overbearing governmental regulations, societal insistence of medical care as a right, and provider constraints all culminate in insurmountable barriers to efficient and effective care.

Presently, legislators have sought solutions by delegating disease-care delivery to industry caretakers with the premise of value-based purchasing of disease care. In other words, value is enhanced through reductions in costs and improvements in outcomes. Unfortunately, the foundation of the American healthcare system remains "fee for service" reimbursement, which incentivizes higher volumes of services per time. But when money is scarce, and pressures to control costs exist, providers and patients are typically the ones who suffer . . . not industry caretakers.

As a result of these developments, the doctor-patient relationship has become less nuanced and far less personal. Both doctors and patients complain to bemused bureaucrats with no answers in sight. Patients have legitimate expectations of receiving quality care, and doctors are under tremendous pressure to provide such care with dwindling amounts of resources. A dichotomy between patient expectations and what providers can offer has developed. Patients expect a healthcare system focused on health rather than disease, while providers remain confined to a system of regulations, laws, and reimbursement structures that remains focused on disease rather than health. Developing a health-centric model of care with the current healthcare system is not only necessary to curb the rising costs of disease-based care, but also is needed to restore critical nuances required for quality individualized care.

Why Is Nuanced Care Important for Physicians?

Under the current "value purchase" model adopted by the various caretakers of healthcare, providers become a commodity rather than a source of innovation. Innovation in healthcare has instead been delegated to pharmaceutical and medical device companies. Despite being the backbone of medicine, medical nuances have progressively taken a backseat over the last fifty years. Medical nuance reflects the art of medicine. It is a provider's mojo or magic charm that leaves patients not only amazed but grateful. The lack of this nuance does not necessarily suggest bad medical care, but its absence does result in a more mundane and mechanical approach to care.

The advances in disease care made over the last century have relied mainly on the insights of engineers and chemists who have been clever enough to find innovative ways to help clinicians establish a diagnosis or cure a disease. Most of the heavy lifting has been done in laboratories all over the world. But such developments are fraught with delays with varying degrees of lag times between laboratory discovery and patient application. The flow of information from the research lab to the clinical arena has been clunky and problematic.

Efforts to translate discoveries and implement relevant solutions to current medical problems have thus been less than ideal. Many of these modern innovations and discoveries, despite their noted benefits, have left most providers by the wayside. Providers are asked to shoulder most of the heavy burden in caring for patients, but for one reason or the other, they have been denied the opportunity to participate in the innovation itself. This lack of opportunity naturally fosters a sense of frustration among providers, as they must navigate a healthcare system that fails to serve the very people for which they took an oath to provide quality care.

The US healthcare system has been based on misdirected incentives for too long. As a result, costs have increased while utilization remains excessive. Therefore, a push for value-based care delivery has come to the forefront. Instead of basing reimbursements on the volume of services provided, linking payments to outcomes has been proposed as a means to change incentives. The focus will naturally shift toward quality of care and efficiency, allowing reduced costs and use of resources. But while this proposal reflects a step in the right direction, it is far from a complete solution.

A focus on quality outcomes for healthcare certainly supports greater value, but still the focus remains on disease rather than health. Health promotion and disease prevention services are warranted as well in order to control costs, more effectively use resources, and optimally promote wellness. Likewise, personalized medicine where providers and patients develop strong healthcare relations can help shift the focus on health promotion and preservation instead of on disease care alone. Nuanced care has the potential to greatly enhance this aspect of healthcare.

Even with a shift in incentives and a more personalized care approach, accessibility and affordability remain key issues. For many, a lack of insurance hinders appropriate care, but even for those with health insurance, out-of-pocket expenses and a lack of coverage for disease prevention measures often exists. Statistically, more than half of all patients with insurance who have chronic illnesses fail to keep preventive appointments, attain needed screening tests, or adhere to medication instructions because of cost factors. In fact, estimates in cost savings for improvements in medication adherence alone are high as $105 billion per year.[1] In order to shift the focus away from disease and toward true health, these issues must be addressed.

Last, measures of quality are often lacking. How can we determine if patients are receiving true quality of care? Such a measure is particularly key for patients with multiple chronic illnesses or conditions. Developing such care measures is important, but waiting for such measures through research pathways is not necessarily practical. Personalized medicine offers the best opportunity to better assess quality of care, and by adopting measures that incentivize this approach, more effective health promotion, disease prevention, and disease management will result.

The development of our current healthcare system has evolved through the course of many decisions and actions, and naturally, different healthcare players will pursue what is in their best interest. Similarly, providers must do the same, using their own ingenuity and the wealth of knowledge they have gained over the years. Through

---

1   Partnership to Fight Chronic Disease (PFCD), "The costly chronic disease epidemic," PFCD website, 2016, http://www.fightchronicdisease.org/sites/default/files/PFCD_WhitePaper_FINAL.pdf.

these efforts, providers will be reminded of the patient care oath they took many years prior, which in turn will motivate them to reclaim the ability to care for patients in a more personal manner based not only on science but also on nuances derived from the art of medicine.

Why Is Nuanced Care Important for Patients?

Patients entrust their physicians to provide the best care possible. For patients, providers represent the face of healthcare. They don't know the names of their health plan's CEO or the names of those who make the bigger decisions regarding their healthcare. They only know the names of their providers, and they rightfully expect quality care from them. But spending more than a few minutes face-to-face with a provider is becoming a rarity. As time has become a limited resource, and as terms like relative value unit (RVU) and full-time equivalents (FTE) have become part of healthcare language, such nuanced care has dwindled.

The effects are quite obvious. Progressively, the focus of care has been on disease management rather than on disease prevention and health promotion. In order to educate and assist patients with positive changes in their lives to promote better health, both time and provider interaction are required. According to the World Health Organization (WHO), more than two-thirds of vascular disorders and cases of diabetes could be prevented through proper diet, exercise, and avoidance of tobacco. The same applies to more than a third of cancer cases.[2] If these goals are to be realized, patients need (and deserve) nuanced care.

Patients often worry about what they eat, the air they breathe, how they slept the night before, and many other things. Patients need time with a provider to not only share these concerns but to also allow

---

2   World Health Organization, "Chronic diseases and health promotion," 2016, http://www.who.int/ chp/chronic_disease_report/part1/en/index11.html.

providers the time to process this information. But with progressive changes in the management of healthcare, opportunities for extended provider-patient rapport have come to a screeching halt. And mediocrity has been the result. Restoring nuance and enabling this rapport is necessary to realize better healthcare and disease management.

Barriers to achieving nuanced care for patients do exist, however. In addition to the healthcare management challenges already noted, there is a shortage of primary care providers in many areas. According to a physician workforce report released in 2016 by the Association of American Medical Colleges, a special analysis showed that if underserved patients had barriers to utilization removed, the United States would need nearly one hundred thousand doctors today to meet patient needs.[3] Even with the addition of physician assistants and nurse practitioners to help fill this void, shortages will remain. And this still fails to address the time limitations involving provider and patient interactions. Clearly, developing the means to restore personalized, nuanced care to medicine will require a dedicated effort by all of society.

Why Is Nuanced Care Important for Society?

Rising healthcare costs, changing population demographics, dwindling healthcare resources, and accessibility barriers represent only a few of the major hurdles facing healthcare today. Determining how to address these areas while focusing on quality of care and a patient-centric perspective is certainly challenging. But developing solutions remains important. The quality of one's healthcare directly impacts one's perceived quality of life. And all communities throughout the world face similar challenges in healthcare. As a result, solutions will

---

3   M. J. Dill and E. S. Salsberg, "The Complexities of Physician Supply and Demand: Projections through 2025, 2008," *Association of American Medical Colleges: Center for Workforce Studies: Washington DC* (2014): 1–94.

not only impact specific nations or regions but global health as well.

One potential solution involves the use of technologies. Advances in information technology (IT) provide robust health monitoring and delivery systems that can be patient centric while also bypassing healthcare barriers. Likewise, technologies can enhance knowledge through information access and encourage more effective choices by patients and providers alike. Information technologies can even expedite the translation of research findings into clinical practice.

Interestingly, most of the decisions that affect healthcare take place outside the medical system. Poor health often involves many factors related to housing, transportation, food security, and other socioeconomic stresses. The healthcare system can be more effective and more efficient if it considers resources available outside the medical system that support improved health. Engaging and collaborating with community-based organizations, public health agencies, and social services can greatly expand healthcare resources. Likewise, encouraging people to be more directly involved in their overall health and well-being taps into additional avenues of support.

Primary healthcare providers (physicians, physician assistants, nurses, pharmacists, and other clinicians) are instrumental in delivering preventive services and encouraging healthy behaviors. Unfortunately, the healthcare system is not organized in a way that fully supports these behaviors. New payment models must assure access to high-quality care, emphasize improving patient health outcomes, reduce costs and wastes, and allow for continued innovation while supporting personalized care for patients. Improvement in these areas is essential in order to facilitate a transition from an acute care, disease-focused model to one focused on prevention, early detection, and health promotion.

Nuanced care benefits communities, societies, and the world at large. With more personalized care, prevention and health promotion efforts are better realized, and the utilization of all available resources becomes increasingly likely. Through these efforts, populations become healthier, which in turn reduces healthcare costs and disease burden while enhancing economic productivity and overall quality of life. Nuanced care not only provides benefits to individuals and providers, but it also aids all of society.

Leading the Way

Providers are entrusted for their skill, compassion, and abilities in providing quality health to their patients. Intuitively, then, providers should be actively involved in designing the future architecture of the healthcare system. Armed with a knowledge of healthcare and the needs of patients, providers are much better equipped to guide the process of change than their business counterparts. Team approaches and interdisciplinary collaboration will be essential tools in delivering optimal healthcare in the future. Wellness-oriented teams of professionals offer great promise in bringing innovation and creative solutions to the table. Providers will naturally lead in this regard, given their skills and expertise.

The US healthcare system has always been recognized for its scope and pace of innovation and discovery. But continued progress in these areas in the future depends upon the existence of an environment that encourages and rewards advances in detection, treatment, and care delivery. In order to achieve such an environment, access to information is essential. Fortunately, the tools exist today to facilitate this access, and through IT solutions, providers can better develop effective strategies for healthcare.

Giving healthcare providers accurate, timely information at the point of care facilitates the delivery of the highest quality, evidence-based medicine. By supporting more effective coordination of care and by ensuring access to patient and clinical information across a delivery system, all healthcare efforts can be enhanced. This not only includes disease management but prevention and health promotion services as well. In order to achieve this goal, health IT must be seamless (interoperable, accessible, usable) wherever the patient obtains services.

Including the patient in this process is important. Facilitating Americans' ability to track their own health and to obtain information on specific conditions and treatment options at the point of decision making is required for patient-centric care. Electronic health records (EHRs) and personal health records (PHRs) can provide patients with valuable information, and foster collaborative care that includes self-management. But the benefits of EHRs and PHRs depend on their ease of accessibility and use by the patient. This reflects yet another nuance of care to consider.

The aforementioned issues become even more important when dealing with patients with multiple conditions. Patients with chronic illnesses who see many providers, take multiple prescription medicines, and require complex monitoring need proactive and collaborative management. Connecting providers with public and private health systems through enhanced interoperability facilitates these goals through information sharing and access to disease registries. Likewise, such efforts can provide many healthcare stakeholders, including patients, with knowledge on ongoing research and clinical trials relevant to their conditions. With these IT tools now available, the time has come for providers to once again take the lead in constructing the future of healthcare. Through these efforts, healthcare can once again become more personalized and individualized so quality care is efficient and effective.

Coalescing around an Idea

The idea of a health-centric healthcare system compared to a disease-centric model reflects a total paradigm shift when envisioning twenty-first-century healthcare. Current state-of-the-art information technology and the ikioo remote health monitoring and management system allow for such accommodations. Providers and patients can align their efforts for a health-focused quality outcome. This does not mean disease care or existing effective practices are abandoned, but it does emphasize a shift in focus from illness to health.

Healthcare workforce shortages are well documented and compromise access to care, particularly in underserved areas. Many in the healthcare workforce (such as pharmacists, patient liaisons, and community health workers) are underutilized and could help to fill these gaps. Greater information sharing and the removal of care barriers could improve adherence to treatment algorithms. And comprehensive prevention, early detection, and cost-sharing approaches among various disease management resources could help provide key solutions to current healthcare system challenges.

Consumers must have easy access to understandable information about health insurance plans and intervention decisions, and also information on lifestyle choices and participation in disease-screening efforts. Community-based programs today provide aging-in-place services, disease management coaching, and preventive care services in lower cost settings with proven results. Integrating these services more closely with the healthcare system through information sharing and patient empowerment can increase support for patients and their families while reducing healthcare costs.

Providers and patients can coalesce around this paradigm shift in healthcare that embraces a patient-centric and health-focused model within the current framework and norms of medical practice. Predictive medical information technology is still in its infancy, but these technologies offer tremendous potential for improving healthcare. Personalized nuanced care can be realized through the use of these technologies and enhanced by embedding predictive machine learning in the process. Such opportunities offer providers a chance to recapture the art of medicine while serving as the change agents needed for radical innovation in healthcare.

CHAPTER 2

Twentieth-Century Healthcare

The current US healthcare system is one of the most complicated ones in the world. Because the system has been established on a fee-for-service model and has since undergone many reforms, its complexities are often difficult to comprehend. In addition, it has evolved into a system with inherent inefficiencies. In an effort to better understand how the current healthcare system has developed over time, a description of current structures, regulations, and challenges will be addressed in an effort to not only appreciate its current state but to envision directions for future change.

Stakeholders in US Healthcare

The US healthcare system is complex in both structure and in the way it functions. Numerous stakeholders exist within healthcare, including patients, providers, hospitals, and the public, as well as private insurers. Interestingly, however, each stakeholder has a different agenda, and each views healthcare differently as well. As a result, pressures to change the system can vary depending on the point of view.

Being the majority stakeholder and ultimate arbiter, the US government focuses on quality care with an emphasis on cost effectiveness, accessibility, efficiency, and a level playing field. On the other hand, providers strive to deliver better care with the latest evidence-based, peer-reviewed innovations. Unfortunately, many of these newer interventions are expensive, and many providers feel the need to practice defensive medicine by using the most advanced technologies. As a result, overall expenditures can become excessive while limited resources are utilized inefficiently. The conflicting interests between the government and providers are readily apparent.

A patient typically seeks any care that meets or exceeds expectations according to the perceived standards of care. However, this standard and level of expectation varies both over time and from place to place. As legal cases and rewards for medical negligence have increased, expectations have similarly advanced. Last, hospitals and healthcare insurers tend to pursue profitable care, ensuring revenues exceed costs. While hospitals align their efforts with their mission statements, they inherently focus on the business of healthcare, as do insurers. Thus, depending on which stakeholder one considers, the area of attention and ultimate goal of healthcare can vary.

With so many players in the healthcare game, fragmentation is inevitable. But fragmentation does have some benefits. Healthcare fragmentation has led to increases in research and innovation. Likewise, scalability, robustness, and level of quality have similarly increased as well. But fragmentation has led to marked inefficiencies and rising costs. In fact, the US spends approximately double the amount per capita on healthcare than the next highest nation in the world. For these reasons, no other healthcare system is comparable to the American healthcare system.

The Structure of the US Healthcare System

The healthcare sector in the US is naturally a major player in the economy, and as a result, millions of individuals are employed within this industry. Nearly fifteen million healthcare providers and allied health professionals work in the healthcare sector. This not only includes doctors and nurses but also therapists, dentists, pharmacists, and administrators. And as noted, each has unique interests and perspectives.[4]

Each of these professionals must be educated and trained in order to have the skills necessary to render quality healthcare services. Altogether, more than three hundred medical schools, dental schools, and pharmacy programs exist currently in the US. This pales to the number of nursing programs in the US, which is approximately five times this figure. And given the number of classes within these curriculums, the demand for educators and administrators within these programs is staggering. In fact, some of these programs predict a shortage of supply of the needed personnel to train providers in the future as healthcare demands rise.[5]

While the percentage of the population involved in healthcare is tremendous, the necessary infrastructure needed to provide healthcare services is even more impressive. The number of acute-care hospitals approximates six thousand in the country, with more than thirty-five million admissions and discharges each year. Likewise, nearly thirty thousand nursing homes, mental health hospitals, and home healthcare agencies exist in the US. And these figures fail to consider the number of outpatient provider offices, diagnostic centers, and public health clinics scattered throughout every community in the nation.[6]

How is this massive system financed? Despite millions of people lacking access and health insurance in America, the vast majority have health insurance to help cover medical expenses. Roughly a third of individuals have government health insurance such as Medicare, Medicaid, or other less common federal or state programs, while another half have employer-sponsored health insurance through private health insurances. And among these private insurers, various products

---

4   Leiyu Shi and Douglas A. Singh, *Essentials of the U.S. Health Care System* (Jones & Bartlett Publishers, 2015).

5   HRSA, 2016.

6   Shi, 2015.

such as health maintenance organizations (HMOs), preferred provider organizations (PPOs), and exclusive provider organizations (EPOs) may be offered at different prices. The remainder of individuals either lack coverage, self-insure, or acquire their own private insurance outside of their employer.[7]

With the aforementioned system in place, healthcare coverage seemingly offers adequate protections for most Americans. But the costs involved with these various healthcare coverage products are tremendous. In fact, healthcare spending has now exceeded 17 percent of the nation's gross domestic product (GDP). In other words, we pay more than a sixth of what we produce simply for healthcare services. The proportion of taxes going to government-funded programs has risen sharply over several decades, and both out-of-pocket costs and premiums for private health insurance have risen as well. Pressures are mounting to contain expenditures while still negotiating adequate care and access.

In considering healthcare structures, three cornerstones are often highlighted. These include costs, quality, and accessibility. Many times these three facets compete with one another. For example, higher quality often means the use of a higher number of services or more advanced technologies, thus raising healthcare costs. Likewise, as healthcare costs rise, insurers must raise premiums to cover these costs, and access to healthcare coverage for some will decline. However, these three areas are not always in competition. Through efficiency and innovation, higher quality at lower costs is achievable, notably when existing inefficiencies exist. Also, broader access to prevention services and health promotion can also lower costs and raise health quality. Thus, while the US is facing serious economic pressures to reform its healthcare system, opportunities as well as challenges do exist.[8]

---

7   Ibid.
8   David Hyman, ed., *Improving Healthcare: A Dose of Competition*, vol. 9, Springer Science & Business Media, 2007.

One of the most significant issues related to achieving these goals relates to the increase in chronic disease care in the US. Currently, the top 5 percent of the population receiving healthcare services accounts for about half of all healthcare expenditures. And the majority of these individuals suffer from various chronic health conditions like diabetes, arthritis, obesity, and heart failure. These types of conditions not only result in costs from direct care services, but also for sizable indirect costs such as lost wages. And with the aging of society, due to baby boomers reaching older age and increasing longevity, the prevalence of chronic diseases is expected to rise even further. Unfortunately, the fragmented nature of the US healthcare system is unable to effectively accommodate these needs. Meeting additional healthcare demands based on the existing system will clearly be unsustainable.[9]

While chronic disease and the aging population exert cost pressures on society, other pressures come from how society views healthcare. In fact, healthcare is often described as a special type of consumer good. Under normal market situations, consumers have access to adequate information about the products and services they want, allowing them to make decisions about price and purchasing, thus affecting demand. However, the healthcare system doesn't work this way. Not only is the system insulated from consumer demand based on regulations and defined fee structures, but consumers likewise have insufficient information about health and healthcare overall to make informed decisions. As a result, consumers rely on the suppliers of these services (doctors, dentists, pharmaceutical companies, hospitals, etc.) to be a surrogate for interpreting this information in a fair and honest way. While the majority of suppliers attempt to be honest purveyors of information, these interpretations still fall short when compared to a free market situation.[10]

---

9   J. Gerteis, D. Izrael, D. Deitz, L. LeRoy, R. Ricciardi, T. Miller, and J. Basu, "Multiple chronic conditions chartbook," *Rockville, MD: Agency for Healthcare Research and Quality (AHRQ) Publications* (2014).
10   Hymen, 2007.

Healthcare is a special good in another way. Unlike other products and services in which consumers are expected to pay for what they receive, this is not always the case for healthcare. For someone with an emergent illness, a level of expectation exists within society that providers will care for him or her. Likewise, negative sentiments often exist when high insurance premiums restrict adequate access to healthcare. While the structure of the healthcare system supports healthcare as a privilege and not an inherent right, feelings are present that support the opposite. Like public education, healthcare is often seen as a basic necessity that society should provide. However, the historical structure of the American healthcare system conflicts with these feelings.[11]

The last consideration regarding America's healthcare structure relates to the multiple agents involved in paying for healthcare services. Ultimately, consumers pay for healthcare services since taxes fund government-based healthcare, wage reductions support employer-based coverage, and direct premiums and copays by individuals are involved in other private insurance options. But each of these insurers (or agents) does not typically communicate with one another. As a result, each has their own set of administrative costs related to healthcare, and each interacts with healthcare providers in different ways. As a result, these multiple agents contribute to healthcare fragmentation and the resultant inefficiency and higher costs.[12]

This overview of the US healthcare structure helps highlight both its complexities as well as the pressures it faces. Certainly, resource constraints and rising expenditures pose major issues, as do the rise in chronic disease and the demand for universal access. But at the same time, several areas for improvement exist. Opportunities include enhanced consumer decision making through better information access, and the ability to reduce fragmentation and improve efficiencies.

---

11   Ibid.
12   Ibid.

Before directly addressing these issues, however, we'll take a deeper look into the US payer system for healthcare.

The Evolution of Today's Healthcare Payment Systems

The US healthcare system is among one of the most complicated systems in the world. The reason for its complex nature has a great deal to do with its historical development over time. Unlike healthcare systems of other countries, the US had some unique developments throughout its evolution that play a significant role in the current system today. By detailing these various changes to the system, we can better appreciate today's complicated payment systems. We will discuss various payers and stakeholders as each relates to the overall healthcare payment system.

For the most part, the majority of Americans have some type of healthcare coverage. But a persistent segment of the population lacks health insurance and thus access to adequate healthcare. Prior to the Affordable Care Act, between forty and fifty million people were uninsured. With expansion of Medicare and the creation of health insurance exchanges, this figure has dropped, but a sizable number of people still fall through the coverage cracks. And this segment typically drives up healthcare expenditures since lack of insurance coverage is associated with absence of preventive measures, a lack of regular healthcare services, and more adverse health conditions.[13] Therefore, while advances in payment systems have improved in some aspects, universal coverage is still not reality at this time.

In subsequent sections, we will discuss employer-based payment systems, private commercial insurance payers, and government-based payers. In addition, we will cover reactions of various stakeholders and providers to regulatory and insurance-based changes in relation to their effects on healthcare payment systems. Most of the changes that

---

13   Ibid.

have shaped the current US healthcare payment system have occurred within the latter half of the twentieth century. Therefore, we must understand these changes in order to appreciate today's healthcare issues and payment strategies.

Employer-Based Insurance Payments

Today's healthcare payment system is a direct reflection of historical changes over the course of time. Interestingly, the initial payment system evolved after World War II and into the 1950s. During that time, employers needed to attract workers to their companies, and labor unions were able to negotiate better work conditions. As a result, health insurance offered by employers became a key bargaining tool. And while this is not the only source of health coverage today, the US healthcare system remains strongly entrenched in an employer-based healthcare model.[14]

Employer-based health insurance coverage can be structured in a variety of ways. Commonly, employers utilize private commercial insurance carriers to administer and provide health insurance coverage to their employees and sometimes retirees. Depending on employer size, varying degrees of leverage may exist in negotiating costs and offerings of different health insurance plans. Alternatively, employers may also choose to develop self-funded health plans for their employees. These plans may be ideal for larger organizations or those operating within healthcare systems, but often the costs and challenges of administering and developing such plans are prohibitive. As a result, some employers may opt for a combination health plan where health insurance is self-funded but the company contracts with a commercial insurance payer to administer the plan and contract with health providers.[15]

---

14   Shi, 2015.
15   Hymen, 2007.

In general, six of every ten individuals in the US has employ-er-based health insurance coverage. Its presence varies by market sector and by the number of employees a firm has. While historical events shaped employer-based coverage prevalence, continued feder-al subsidies have perpetuated its popularity. Specifically, employers who provide such coverage are able to deduct costs from corporate taxes, and the benefits received are not considered as taxable income to employees. Thus, employer-based health insurance is purchased with pretax dollars. While this structure helps both employer and employee, ultimately employees bear the highest burden of health insurance costs in this situation.[16] As strategies to maximize company profits are pursued, the costs of healthcare insurance coverage are shifted to employees through reduced wage growth over time.

Medicare and Medicaid Payments

In addition to employer-based insurance coverage, the mid-1960s brought about government social reforms that resulted in the creation of Medicare and Medicaid. Medicare was established to ensure that adults age sixty-five years and older had health insurance coverage, and this has since been expanded to include children with disabilities as well as individuals with end-stage renal disease and amyotrophic lateral sclerosis. Medicaid, on the other hand, was a state-based program supplemented with federal funding to provide healthcare services for low-income individuals. Given the sizable populations these entitlement programs serve, it is understandable that they remain a pillar of the healthcare payment system.[17] In fact, both programs continue to expand.

The initial Medicare and Medicaid payment systems were relatively straightforward. For Medicare, Part A provided coverage for hospital

16   Ibid.
17   Ibid.

services, and hospitals were paid according to their actual costs. However, no incentives to lower costs were initially present, so hospitals' expenditures remained high. At the same time, incentives for consumers to be selective about hospitals services were lacking as well. Thus, hospital stays and use of services skyrocketed. And because Medicare Part A was funded through payroll taxes paid by both employers and employees, increases in Medicare costs eventually meant increases in payroll taxes.[18] The negative economic impacts resulting from this are considerable.

While Part A covered hospital services, Medicare Part B covered physician services and diagnostics. Unlike Part A, Part B was financed through general federal funds, and therefore, various tax revenues supported this component of Medicare. Under a fee-for-service system, Medicare initially reimbursed physicians according to their standard and customary fees charged. And similar to hospital reimbursements, no incentives for efficiency or cost containment existed for physicians or patients. As expected, the result has been significant increases in expenditures for Medicare Part B as well.[19]

Medicaid was established with federal standards in place, but states were responsible for determining eligibility criteria and coverage for specific populations. In general, Medicaid offers healthcare services for low-income individuals who have incomes below 133 percent of the federal poverty line. Likewise, it also provides services for children and women in specific situations, as well as a bulk of long-term care services. In total, more than fifty million Americans are covered primarily by Medicaid insurance. Similar to Medicare programs, however, Medicaid did not provide incentives for cost-efficient care, and it too placed a burden on state revenues. Given the sizable populations that Medicare and Medicaid covered, before long, rising healthcare expenditures stimulated reforms.

---

18   Ibid.
19   Ibid.

While government insurance programs covered select groups, private health insurers offered coverage to others. These companies provided coverage for both employers and individuals, and their initial packages were based on a fee-for-service system. In other words, a patient receiving a provider service paid the fee associated with that service. This fee was paid regardless of the quality of the care provided or the outcome. Likewise, providers initially established their own fees rather than having to negotiate fee schedules with payers. However, as healthcare expenditures began to rise, this system changed dramatically.[20]

Through the 1970s and 1980s, both private insurers and government payers began to pursue measures to control healthcare costs. For government programs, fees for physician provider services were reduced while a diagnostic related group (DRG) system was developed for hospitals to contain payments for specific conditions. Private insurance companies followed suit, developing a number of managed care options to control costs. Provider fees were now negotiated to reduce expenditures, and the allowable number of services was restricted. Providers naturally met these changes with resistance, and likewise consumers also reluctantly accepted the changes. Despite managed care resulting in reduced premiums for consumers, many could no longer access their provider of choice or the services they desired.[21]

One of the major changes that took place during this time involved the progressive shift from a fee-for-service model to a progressive payment system. In fee-for-service models, payment is determined retrospectively based on the number and types of services provided. Providers are incentivized to provide more services, and consumers to consume more with no incentive for efficiency, quality, or cost containment. The fee-for-service payment structures combined with health insurance protections and a lack of consumer knowledge about

---

20   Ibid.
21   Shi, 2015.

healthcare services served to boost utilization. Likewise, providers had no reason to compete based on price of services within this model.[22]

In 1983, Congress chose to abandon the retrospective fee-for-service payment system in favor of prospective payments to providers. In contrast to retrospective payment systems, prospective payment systems determine reimbursement in advance based on diagnoses, conditions, and service packages. The DRG system imposed a pre-determined value of an inpatient stay given the condition for which the patient was admitted. For example, for a patient admitted with heart failure, a hospital would receive a specified amount whether the patient stayed three days or five days. Naturally, this incentivized greater efficiency and lesser use of resources. Likewise, the DRG system took various factors into consideration for some hospitals that served more complicated or unhealthy populations. Additional outlier payments were included in standard DRG reimbursement rates for some teaching hospitals and hospitals serving low-income areas because of the presumed higher costs related to healthcare services provided. Under the DRG system, not only were fewer inpatient resources used, but fewer overall admissions resulted as well.[23]

Because of these developments, a shift toward greater outpatient care resulted since better reimbursement rewards existed in this healthcare setting. Therefore, it should come as no surprise that government payers adopted an outpatient prospective payment system for hospitals and other care facilities as well. In 2003, an ambulatory payment classification (APC) system was developed by the Centers for Medicare and Medicaid Services, which assigned reimbursement rates for 750 different outpatient services. This outpatient prospective payment system was based on median costs for providing the services, and variations occurred annually based on new data. And

---

22   Ibid.
23   Ibid.

subsequent outpatient prospective payment fees were developed for skilled nursing facilities and home healthcare services as well.[24]

Subsequently, government payers also developed a resource-based relative value scale (RBRVS) for physician services where reimbursement was determined based on regional costs, practice overhead, liability insurance payments, materials, and practice type. Like the DRG and APC systems, RBRVS similarly used cost data to calculate physician reimbursement rates. Thus, instead of hospitals, physicians, and other providers determining their costs and preferred reimbursement, the government began dictating these figures. In some instances, such as inpatient services, utilization benefits were realized as services and lengths of stays diminished. But in other areas, inefficiencies and problems continued. For example, for home healthcare services, prospective payment schedules reduced the number of beneficiaries receiving services as well as the number of services offered. Likewise, for physicians, higher patient volumes were used to offset reductions in reimbursement rates, often at the expense of the patient-provider interaction quality.[25]

Overall, the purchase of healthcare services by government health insurance programs inherently has notable problems. Ideally, reimbursement systems would effectively replicate a competitive market situation, but this is not the case in healthcare. In some instances, Medicare and Medicaid offer higher reimbursement rates for specific services when compared to others. As a result, these services end up occupying a larger segment of the market than would otherwise be the case when services are driven by consumer demand and competition. Also, Medicare and Medicaid may pay too much or too little for specific services. When they pay too much, resources are wasted; and when they pay too little, capacity, quality, and innovation are diminished.

---

24   Hymen, 2007.
25   Ibid.

Historically, both Medicare and Medicaid have focused more on costs than on quality of healthcare services. Prior to the 1990s, little effort was made to reward or punish providers based on the quality of patient outcomes. In the 1990s, some efforts were made to begin reporting quality outcomes in certain areas. Skilled nursing facilities, home healthcare agencies, and hospitals began reporting outcomes, as well as reports on specific conditions and treatments like dialysis for renal disease. Notably, these reports have demonstrated positive effects on mortality rates, and they have shown that provider behaviors are more quality focused when utilized. But such efforts to focus on quality of services have clearly lagged behind policies that seek to limit costs and expenditures.[26]

Over the course of the last several years, the Center for Medicare and Medicaid Services has begun to shift its focus in the direction of quality as well as cost containment. Bundled payments and shared savings programs are being evaluated to assess their ability to enhance patient outcomes while also cutting costs. In essence, these programs reimburse multiple providers under one payment for a condition-related event. Often, these providers may include a hospital, physicians, and even post-acute care entities like home healthcare agencies. In this system, a single payment is provided for all services associated with that condition for a specific number of days, which may range from thirty to ninety days. Providers must then determine which services are provided, which provider provides these services, and how reimbursements are distributed. Estimates suggest that these programs may reduce Medicare expenditures by as much as 10 percent.[27]

By forcing multiple providers to collaborate on patient care in bundled payment programs, fragmentation of healthcare services is reduced. Likewise, providers who are best qualified to provide them,

---

26   Ibid.
27   Dennis Delisle, M. H. S. A. "Big things come in bundled packages: implications of bundled payment systems in health care reimbursement reform," *American Journal of Medical Quality* (2013).

from both a quality and cost perspective, ideally perform the services. Because any negative occurrence or outcome reduces the profits received from the bundled payment, all providers have a strong incentive to provide high quality care at the lowest price. But while this type of system does provide important incentives, inherent problems will likely remain in establishing accurate reimbursement rates for bundled payment determinations.[28]

Many unintended consequences will likely result from this new reimbursement system based on the lack of experience with such programs. For example, some providers may try to shift care into the post-acute care period and beyond as a means to increase their reimbursement. Likewise, up-coding might occur to label patients with higher levels of acuity or severity than they might otherwise have in an effort to maximize reimbursements. And providers may seek to increase the number of patient bundles in an effort to increase income. These are unknowns with the adoption of this new bundled payment system, and the inclusion of other providers in the post-acute care period may have additional effects as well. For example, the determination of when a patient is ready for discharge, transfer, or ultimate release from services may all be affected through these new reimbursement models and their related incentives.[29]

Despite the limitations noted in Medicare and Medicaid health insurance programs, these entities do and will continue to represent a major source of healthcare funding. As a result, understanding how these health insurance programs have evolved over time helps one to appreciate future changes. In addition, both Medicare and Medicaid policy changes have typically been a key driver of changes in employer-based health insurance plans and in private commercial health insurance carrier decisions. Knowing the current direction in

---

28   Ibid.
29   Rand Corporation, "Analysis of bundled payments," *Website*, n.d., http://www.rand.org/pubs/technical_reports/TR562z20/analysis-of-bundled-payment.html.

Medicare and Medicaid is important as a means to assess the overall healthcare market structure.

Private Commercial Health Insurers

As noted, employers have utilized private commercial health insurers in many instances to provide health insurance coverage to their employees. At the same time, many individuals also utilize private health plans to ensure coverage for healthcare services. Estimates in the past have shown that 7 percent of the population under age sixty-five years utilizes this type of health insurance coverage. However, because individuals have less bargaining leverage when compared to large employers, individual insurance coverage rates are generally more costly when compared to employer-based insurance rates. Regardless, this type of health insurance still occupies a significant segment of healthcare payers.[30]

Just as Medicare and Medicaid experienced marked increases in healthcare expenditures in the late 1960s and early 1970s, private commercial insurance carriers did as well. However, legislation triggered some notable changes beginning in 1973. The Health Maintenance Act passed by Congress provided funds for insurers to develop managed care plans to help contain rising healthcare costs. Not only did this legislation override state laws that prohibited managed care organizations, it also required larger-size employers to offer a choice involving a managed care health plan product. As a result, a dramatic change in commercial health plan programs occurred.[31]

Managed care organizations, in essence, strive to integrate the financial and care delivery aspects of healthcare with each type of managed care product, and are successful in varying degrees. Most commonly, consumers have restricted choices regarding providers

---

30   Hymen, 2007.
31   Ibid.

and/or healthcare services in exchange for reduced premiums, copays, and deductibles. Conversely, greater managed care product choice in these areas results in higher consumer payment burdens. With this concept in mind, employers may offer a number of different managed care products, with some of the more common health plan products being health maintenance organization (HMO) plans, preferred provider organization (PPO) plans, and point of service (POS) plans.[32]

Within the various managed care health plan products, different strategies are invoked in an effort to control healthcare spending. The first involves selective provider contracting where only certain providers are offered enrollment into a specific health plan. If such a health plan is attractive because of large consumer/patient pools, providers will often bid more competitively to gain enrollment, resulting in lower provider fees. In addition, managed care organizations may try to reduce healthcare costs by restricting access to services through utilization review. With this strategy, providers evaluate whether a service is medically indicated or necessary before it can be rendered.[33]

Other managed care strategies, such as capitation and financial target rewards, shift risks away from the health insurer. In capitation, providers assume a significant amount of risk when they accept a predetermined payment per patient in advance for a patient population's care over the next quarter or year. In financial target rewards, providers also assume greater risk since financial bonuses or penalties may occur in relation to quality and cost outcomes. Other risk-shifting strategies involve consumers. By varying levels of copays and deductibles, patients can take on lower or higher levels of cost sharing of their care with the health insurer. Depending on the specific product, one or more of these strategies may be used.[34]

Overall, capitation plans are rarely seen today. Many providers failed to appreciate the degree of risk they were assuming, and as a

---

32   Ibid.
33   Ibid.
34   Shi, 2015.

result, some went bankrupt under such payer-provider arrangements. However, HMO and PPO plans remain common, as do many other managed care products. While HMOs require patients to receive primary services through a provider gatekeeper and remain within a specific provider network, PPOs offer greater choice of initial care from a list of preferred providers without such a gatekeeper. POS plans, on the other hand, provide an intermediate level of choice and flexibility by having a primary care gatekeeper but an ability to still see providers who might be out of the plan's network. Depending on the degree of flexibility and choice desired, and the degree of cost a consumer is willing to pay, different managed care plans exist to meet specific needs.[35]

Once RBRVS figures were published for physicians, many commercial insurers used these to determine what they would offer providers as reimbursement. For example, a HMO, which is typically more restrictive in provider and service access, would more closely align payments near the prospective payment system values. PPOs, which were typically less restrictive, would scale their fees slightly higher. Of course, the costs associated with higher reimbursements were passed along to consumers. If a consumer (or employer) wanted the less restrictive PPO plan, then the premiums were higher when compared to a more restrictive HMO plan. Regardless, the ultimate effect of the government prospective payment system was to regulate provider fees across the board, including those from private insurers as well.[36]

Beginning in the late 1990s, managed care began to receive a significant amount of criticism. For one, healthcare expenditures continued to rise, resulting in critiques of administrative costs associated with managed care systems. In addition, many consumers did not like restriction of choice, and providers did not like the second-guessing

---

35   Paul J. Feldstein, *Health Care Economics*, Cengage Learning, 2012.
36   Shi, 2015.

nature of gatekeepers and utilization review. However, objective evidence and surveys demonstrated that quality of care and customer satisfaction of managed care was favorable for the most part. This is likely a reason managed care organizations continue to play a significant role as a US healthcare payer.

Physicians and Physician Group Effects on Payments

As one might expect, physician costs comprise a significant portion of healthcare spending. Past statistics suggest physicians account for 22 percent of all healthcare expenditures. In the 1970s and 1980s, expenditures related to physician costs rose dramatically, averaging a 12 percent increase per year. And even after managed care and RBRVS systems were put into place, physician expenditure rates have continued to increase approximately 5 percent per year.[37] Despite this increase, managed care and government changes have had significant impacts on physician reimbursement and behaviors. While some have reacted in a favorable manner from a competition perspective, others have not.

In response to these pressures, physicians responded in one of two ways. Either they chose to adopt procompetitive strategies to overcome the financial setbacks, or they pursued anticompetitive ones. Those embracing competition offered strategies to lower cost services and deliver higher quality. But others chose to develop collective provider networks to enhance their bargaining position and to exclude competition. For example, independent physician associations (IPAs) consisted of a network of participating physicians that negotiated and approved fee schedules and other parameters in a group. Physician hospital organizations (PHOs) adopted the same strategy, resulting in a joint venture between a hospital system and physicians affiliated with that system.[38]

---

37   Hymen, 2007.
38   Ibid.

The development of various provider networks offered several benefits to providers. In addition to greater collective bargaining power, these networks allowed greater sharing of risk among various stakeholders. While IPAs shared financial and clinical risk among larger numbers of physicians, PHOs did the same between hospital systems and doctors. The result was reduced costs and enhanced clinical efficiency. However, regulatory concerns over antitrust issues were raised. Thus, over time, the benefits of such joint ventures were less effective. Likewise, with a shift away from fee-for-service by government prospective payment programs, negotiations with private insurers made less of an overall impact.[39]

Another type of joint venture that providers pursued was a messenger model. As the name would suggest, a third party conducted negotiations between a health insurance payer and a group of providers. For example, a payer might provide a proposed set of reimbursement schedules for the entire network of providers, and the third party would present these proposals to the network. But unlike other joint ventures, individual providers could choose to accept or reject the proposals without committing the entire network. The benefit of such a system reduced costs related to provider negotiations, and it facilitated negotiation efficiencies. However, like other joint ventures, antitrust violations were likely and could result in serious ramifications.[40]

Unlike other industries, healthcare does not lend itself well to collective bargaining strategies. In general, the government has opposed collective bargaining among physicians because it assumes this will negatively impact consumers. Collective bargaining for higher rates for physician services may result in higher consumer costs and potentially declining quality of care. In fact, some estimates suggest healthcare expenditures could increase between 2 and 3 percent in

---

39   Ibid.
40   Ibid.

such situations. However, physicians argue they should be allowed to collectively bargain since payers have excessive market power within the healthcare sector.[41] This would help level the playing field when it came to fee negotiations. But to date, legislation and rulings have not favored any move in this direction.

One additional area where physicians affect the healthcare system structure relates to credentialing and licensing. In most states, various healthcare professional licensing boards consist of physician members or involve physician oversight. As a result, the ability to restrict not only the number of physicians but also the number of other allied health professionals exists through these licensing and credentialing activities. Notably, this restriction impairs competition significantly, and in turn, often increases costs. Also, these activities can further hinder innovation, as is the case involving telemedicine use and inter-state licensing capacities.[42]

Some physician strategies in dealing with the evolving healthcare system landscape have been effective in achieving better negotiation power and higher quality care. But at the same time, other strategies have undermined innovation and quality advances. As future changes encourage greater provider collaboration and transparency of performance measures, physicians will need to continue to adapt and change. Such changes pose challenges but also provide great opportunities.

Hospitals and Hospital-Related Facility Effects on Payment

Having discussed the effect DRG and prospective payment systems had on hospital systems, it is also noteworthy to consider the effect hospital systems have had on payment structures as well. Like physicians, some hospitals have pursued mergers as a means to enhance their bargaining and negotiation leverage. Initially, hospital mergers

---

41   Ibid.
42   Ibid.

occurred on a much larger scale with national chains of hospitals developing. But over time, the more successful hospital systems have emerged in local and regional areas.

In considering these regional hospital systems, many areas often have a specific hospital that is preferred by consumers in the area. These hospitals have been identified as crucial to private health insurers since including such a hospital may determine whether or not a consumer might choose that insurer's health plans. One effect hospital mergers have had in this regard relates to a significant increase in bargaining ability with health insurers. While insurers have no problem paying higher reimbursement rates for these essential hospitals, they might be reluctant to pay the same rates for other hospitals within the overall hospital system. However, hospital systems often demand the same reimbursement rates among all of their hospitals and not simply the more attractive ones.[43]

Healthcare insurers have tried to combat this tendency by creating a tiered system among hospitals. For instance, a key essential hospital in a region might be labeled a level 3 hospital while a less desirable hospital might be a level 1 or 2. Insurers thus try to carve out different reimbursement rates for services based on the tier level. This strategy encourages consumers to use lower-cost hospitals through cost-sharing strategies, but it also attracts consumers since the essential hospitals are available within their plan. Naturally, hospitals are resistant to such strategies, and they argue creating different tiers for hospitals can falsely label one hospital as providing lower quality care. Depending on the specific region and market, insurers or hospital systems may enjoy a more favorable bargaining position.[44]

Hospital mergers, like joint ventures involving physicians, have been touted as having antitrust concerns. However, judicial cases involving hospital systems have not generally supported such claims to

---

43   Ibid.
44   Ibid.

date. Therefore, hospital mergers tend to be more common and larger in scope than physician joint ventures. In addition, the end result of most hospital mergers has been higher healthcare service prices for both nonprofit and for-profit organizations without any guarantee of greater efficiencies. Thus, on average, it seems hospital mergers have primarily benefitted hospitals without any secondary benefits to consumers or insurer payment structures.

A related development involving hospitals over the last few decades involves single specialty hospitals. Unlike traditional hospitals, single specialty hospitals offer expertise and services in single areas of care. Common examples of such hospitals include those providing specialty care in orthopedics, cardiac care, children's care, and women's health. Interestingly, however, physicians having ownership interest in the facility characterize most of these hospitals. Therefore, these facilities compete directly with traditional hospitals in select areas of care.[45]

Proponents of single-specialty hospitals believe these facilities enhance the quality of care by caring for higher volumes of patients within the specified area of expertise and by utilizing better standards of care. However, opponents suggest that these hospitals choose to care for healthier patients who consume fewer healthcare resources while referring less healthy patients to nearby traditional hospital systems. In fact, traditional hospital systems have responded in some instances by restricting access and privileges of physicians involved in single-specialty hospitals. In other situations, hospitals have chosen to compete by opening up their own single-specialty care wings.[46] In either case, these developments have not made as much of an impact on payment structures as they have on quality aspects of care.

Other facilities that are similar to single-specialty hospitals are ambulatory surgical centers. When patients do not require overnight stays from a surgery, these facilities offer less costly services for the

---

45   Ibid.
46   Ibid.

same procedures when compared to traditional hospital stays. As with other types of healthcare services, Medicare and private insurance reimbursement rates affect the number and types of surgeries considered in these facilities. But without question, consumer convenience and reduced costs are clear benefits of ambulatory surgery centers. And similar to the case with single-specialty hospitals, hospitals have responded in both pro- and anticompetitive ways. While some have opened up their own outpatient ambulatory surgical centers to compete on price and quality, others have restricted access of physicians based on their participation in these facilities.[47]

Throughout the 1990s and into the current era, hospitals and other organizations have sought to both employ physicians and purchase physician practices as a means to achieve better efficiencies, improve system integrations, achieve better patient care management, and better position themselves for new bundled payment reimbursement systems. Though not all of these efforts have been successful, these pursuits did place greater emphasis on quality and value of care while also promoting the use of HITs. However, many physicians have not been supportive of this type of strategy. In the Physician Foundation survey, nearly two-thirds of all physicians did not feel physician employment by hospitals resulted in better quality and lower costs. And half felt the trend of such employment resulted in positive benefits.[48]

One negative effect of physician employment is the increase in physician turnover and detrimental effects to continuity of patient care. Changes in financial and emotional incentives can result in reduced barriers to pursue other sources or positions of employment. In fact, some reports estimate the physician turnover rate among hospital-employed physicians to be as high as 14 percent.[49] Notably, this turnover

---

47 Ibid.
48 T. Singleton and P. Miller, "The Physician Employment Trend: What You Need to Know," *Family Practice Management* 22, no. 4 (2015): 11.
49 Ibid.

adversely affects both physicians and hospitals. Thus, the goals that may be pursued by such arrangements may be undermined by these realities.

Other aspects of the Physician Foundation survey suggested such employment models also negatively affect primary care physician services. Between 2008 and 2014, the average number of patients physicians saw per day dropped by 17 percent under this model of care. Likewise, the average number of hours primary care physicians worked in this setting fell by 6 percent during this same time period. Extrapolating this data into actual physician numbers, this would be the equivalent of losing roughly 45,000 primary care physicians. The reductions, while related in part to physician turnover, were also due to reduced work volumes. Set schedules and reduced financial incentives result in physicians seeing almost two fewer patients per day when comparing employed physicians to independent physicians.[50]

Other differences between employed physicians and independent practitioners are more subjective. Both groups report some frustrations in having adequate clinical autonomy. However, concern exists that employed physicians may have a reduced level of interest in taking ownership of their patients' health outcomes and fully embracing patient advocacy roles. The employment of physicians calls into question whether future doctors have a true professional calling as opposed to being trained technical workers. Other secondary effects may not only undermine certain goals but also bring about larger undesirable changes.[51]

Overall, hospital changes over time have resulted in both positive and negative effects on payment structures in healthcare. Mergers have generally resulted in higher costs and better leverage in fee negotiations while quality of care has not really changed. In other situations, advancing competition from physicians has encouraged

50　Ibid.
51　Ibid.

some cost reductions in services when hospitals choose to compete. Also, organizations (usually consisting of hospitals) have sought to purchase groups of hospitals in an effort to consolidate purchases, resulting in better economies of scale. But when compared to the effects of government and private commercial insurers, hospital systems have had a much lower impact in payment structures in the recent past.

Pharmaceutical Effects on Payment Systems

Historically, patent protections have existed for pharmaceuticals, which have been beneficial to the healthcare system in many ways. First, patents require manufacturers to reveal many aspects of their product, and in doing so, key information becomes available to facilitate other producers to develop other, more advanced pharmaceutical products. In other words, patents in disseminating product information encourage ongoing pharmaceutical innovation. At the same time, the protections offered by patents similarly encourage new product development as well as research since investments are less likely to be thwarted through competition.[52]

While patent protection is important, the effect this has on pharmaceutical pricing can be unwelcome. In order to pay for advanced research and development of both successful and failed drug trials, newly patented drugs are commonly high in price and contribute to increased healthcare expenditures. However, once the patent expires, generic manufacturers can then produce the drug at much lower costs. In 1984, Congress passed the Hatch-Waxman Act, which encouraged competition among generic pharmaceutical manufacturers. This further promoted lower-priced medications, while the patent system continued to promote innovation.[53] Thus, the effects on healthcare payments overall from this perspective have been favorable.

---

52   Ibid.
53   Ibid.

More recent changes within the pharmaceutical arena that may affect payment systems involve third-party entities and advertising changes. Pharmacy benefit managers and mail order pharmacy companies have been used to facilitate efficiency and utilize higher volume pricing discounts. While drug costs are often lower for consumers, it is not yet clear whether third-party players increase administrative costs overall or lower total costs. The allowance of direct consumer advertising has also been controversial in terms of costs. Many suspected such advertising would result in higher utilization of pharmaceuticals and thus raise healthcare spending. But currently evidence is lacking in this regard. Instead, it appears such advertising is a good means by which consumers can be educated about medications, and this in turn may lower utilization in some areas.

For the most part, payments related to pharmaceuticals represent a minority of healthcare expenditures when compared to other areas. Likewise, recent strategies and legislation have promoted opportunities for medication discounts through generic drug production and high-volume pricing. Manufacturers often subsidize high-priced, brand-name pharmaceuticals for individuals who lack adequate funds to purchase needed drugs as well.[54] As a result, this area of healthcare is perhaps of lesser concern when it comes to healthcare payment problems in comparison to other aspects.

The Affordable Care Act

The Essentials of the ACA

In 2010, the Patient Protection and Affordable Care Act (ACA) was established as legislation ushering in a new era in healthcare coverage and access for America. The legislation, though controversial, was an effort to improve the United States' dismal record in healthcare over

---

54   Ibid.

the last several decades. In comparison to other wealthy, developed nations, America is ranked among the last in life expectancy, despite the US having nearly double the amount of expenditures on healthcare overall. Issues concerning cost control, quality improvements, as well as coverage and access to healthcare have been the key areas of focus in considering healthcare reform. The ACA, despite criticisms that the legislation addresses only the accessibility aspect of healthcare, actually addresses all three of these areas.[55]

Significant gaps exist within the US population in terms of health insurance coverage, with large numbers of individuals without healthcare insurance. As of 2013, 15 percent of Americans lacked any health insurance coverage at all. While Medicare and Medicaid programs provide access and coverage for the healthcare of children, the elderly, the disabled, and the significantly impoverished, adults outside of these categories are left without government protections. These individuals, if they are unemployed or lack resources to afford private insurance, often lack health insurance coverage altogether.[56] As a result, millions go without healthcare, and when healthcare needs become urgent, more expensive care is provided through more expensive settings like emergency rooms. This type of care is not only more costly with lower quality outcomes, but it also increases the rate of medical bankruptcy for these individuals.[57]

Often labeled as Obamacare by news media and politicians alike, the ACA was passed, providing measures to move toward universal healthcare coverage for all Americans. Despite universal healthcare coverage having bipartisan support over the last several decades, various groups have become entrenched either for or against Obamacare. Proponents support the legislation, claiming it will reduce healthcare

55   Stephen Zuckerman and John Holahan, "Despite Criticism, The Affordable Care Act Does Much to Contain Healthcare Costs," Urban Institute Health Policy Center, 2012.
56   Jeri A. Milstead, *Health Policy and Politics: A Nurse's Guide* (Jones & Bartlett Learning, 2004).
57   Zuckerman, 2012.

costs, increase accessibility, and improve quality of care while promoting advances in the general welfare of the country. Opponents, on the other hand, claim nearly the opposite, stating Obamacare results in rising healthcare costs, reduced quality of services, and a government takeover of private choice. Without question, the legislation has provoked both debate and controversy.[58]

The ACA went into effect primarily in 2014, requiring individuals to purchase or acquire health insurance or face subsequent taxation penalties. This has become known as the individual mandate. As part of Obamacare, each state was responsible for developing health insurance exchanges through which a number of health insurance companies would offer various insurance coverage policies. However, Obamacare required these plans to have specific requirements, and preventive care was an important one. In addition, health insurance companies could not deny insurance to anyone based on preexisting conditions, gender, or health status. These aspects of the ACA were established to reduce healthcare premiums, improve equity and access for coverage, and enhance quality health outcomes through prevention. These represented major goals of the ACA, important for individuals as well as for the nation as a whole.[59]

Access was a key priority regarding this piece of legislation. The ACA sought to make an immediate impact on individual healthcare insurance coverage by extending Medicaid coverage to those at 138 percent of the federal poverty line and below. In addition, the creation of health insurance exchanges sought to offer affordable insurance coverage to those exceeding this level of income at various cost-sharing levels. These levels include bronze, silver, gold, and platinum tiers of health insurance products. Individuals are now required to

---

58   E. Klein, "The Republicans Turn Against Universal Health Insurance," *The Washington Post*, 2012, http://www.washingtonpost.com/blogs/wonkblog/wp/2012/06/30/the-republican-turn-against-universal-health-insurance/.

59   David Straus, "Managing Healthcare Spending in the United States," *The Journal of Global Health Care Systems* 2, no. 1 (2012).

purchase health insurance from health insurance exchanges or in the private market, or they will be penalized a tax fee annually. This individual mandate went into effect in 2014 as well.[60]

The individual mandate of the ACA has been subsidized in several ways. First, individuals who have fallen under 138 percent of the poverty line are deemed eligible for Medicaid coverage, which alleviates some coverage barriers for low-income individuals. Second, individuals over 138 percent of the poverty line and up to 400 percent are eligible for partial government subsidies, which are to be used to purchase coverage through the health insurance exchanges. But for those earning incomes over 400 percent of the poverty level, expectations are that these individuals will purchase their own insurance coverage. If not, a taxation penalty will be assessed which equals $195 or 1 percent of a person's income, whichever is greater. These penalties are planned to be increased in subsequent years.[61]

Despite these subsidies and entitlements, partial payments for health insurance for some individuals and full payments for others will still be an additional burden consumers have not previously experienced. Initial estimates suggested that as many as twenty-three million individuals will still fall through gaps in ACA policies because they fail to meet criteria for subsidies yet also have too few resources to afford health insurance. The ACA also does nothing to address the millions of undocumented immigrants in the country who still utilize emergency services acutely and fail to have preventive services.[62] Therefore, despite efforts to maximize equity of access, the ACA still has significant limitations.

The ACA, in essence, sought to build upon the existing private healthcare insurance system by including private health insurance

---

60   Zuckerman, 2012.

61   Ibid.

62   M. Boot, "ObamaCare and American Power," *Wall Street Journal*, March 25, 2010, http://www.naegele.com/documents/MaxBoot-ObamaCareandAmericanPower.pdf.

companies in state health insurance exchanges. This plan was implemented in order to allow individuals to keep their existing coverage
and their existing providers. However, insurance providers meeting
exchange qualifications have been limited, and as a result, many individuals have been faced with changing both insurances and providers.
Also, some small businesses that employ fewer than fifty employees
chose to forego health insurance coverage for their employees. This
forced many individuals into the public exchanges who previously
had company-based insurance coverage.[63] These shortcomings of the
ACA have undermined some of the quality measures it has strived to
achieve.

The primary cost savings from the individual mandate are believed
to relate to economies of scale. As larger numbers of people enroll in
health insurance coverage, the costs of healthcare are more widely
distributed, resulting in lower costs per individual. This is further
aided by the requirement for health insurance companies to provide
many preventive services. In theory, this enlarged participation in
the healthcare system should reduce the high cost of premiums since
everyone will now have some obligation to participate. In contrast,
those with health insurance in the past bore the majority of the cost
burden for millions of uninsured individuals by having to pay higher
premiums.[64]

Pooled resources and economies of scale, however, are not accepted
as valid by many opponents of the ACA. Some suspect that while
insurance premiums will be less due to enhanced competition among
insurance companies in the exchanges, the total costs to individuals
will not change significantly. In other cost areas, such as medications
and medical equipment, consumers will pay higher costs, as insurance

---

63   Zuckerman, 2012.
64   S. Fabricant, "Access to Healthcare for the Poor: Will the Affordable Care Act Address Income-Re-
lated Health Disparities in the United States?" *Independent Study Project (ISP) Collection,* Paper 1308,
2012, http://digitalcollections.sit.edu/isp_collection/1308.

companies will refuse to subsidize these costs. In addition, the greater amount of government subsidies to extend Medicaid and to provide partial support for insurance purchases will result in higher taxes for citizens, negating any cost savings from the ACA. And without tort reform, which now encourages the practice of expensive and wasteful defensive medicine, costs for individuals will continue to be higher than they should be.[65]

A second concern of the ACA in relation to individuals is whether it will enhance equity and access of healthcare. Based on extensions of Medicaid and the individual mandate requirements, certainly access will be increased. However, millions will still fall through the gaps in the policies and fail to receive coverage. In addition, healthcare will be far from equitable for many, as different levels of coverage will be offered based on price. This will again result in a rationing of care based on the ability to pay rather than a true universal healthcare coverage. And though the ACA builds upon the existing private healthcare insurance system, many individuals will lose access to their preferred providers.[66]

In addition to the individual mandates, employer mandates were also included in the ACA. For employers with fifty or more employees, healthcare insurance coverage is mandatory for all full-time employees. Naturally, concerns exist that small business employers with fewer employees would forego health insurance, and indeed some have. However, the ACA does incentivize health insurance coverage for employees here as well. For small business owners, tax credits are provided which can allow them to receive up to half of their employee coverage costs. The employer mandate went into effect in 2015, and like individuals, employers also utilize the healthcare exchanges in accessing approved and affordable coverage for their employees.[67]

---

65   M. D. Tanner, "Perils of Obamacare: The Three Big Lies," *CATO Institute*, July 21, 2009, http://www.cato.org/publications/commentary/perils-obamacare-three-big-lies.

66   Fabricant, 2012.

67   Feldstein, 2012.

As mentioned, the ACA enhanced access to coverage by preventing health insurance companies from discriminating against individuals based on their gender, health status, or age. Additionally, a person can no longer be dropped from their insurance plan or charged more for a preexisting condition. In fact, except for the case where fraudulent activities have been documented, the ACA prevents anyone from being terminated from their coverage as long as they make payments. And the ACA eliminated the ability for health insurance companies to impose limits on annual benefits or lifetime rewards as in the past. These limits previously accounted for the bulk of medical bankruptcies in the nation, but as of today, this is no longer allowed.[68]

Other areas where access to health insurance coverage was enhanced involved early retirees and young adults. In terms of early retirees, a re-insurance program was developed for employers to help offer coverage to these workers until the healthcare exchanges were fully developed. Likewise, individuals under the age of twenty-six years could be included on their parents' insurance plans according to the ACA. This group specifically reflected a large number of the uninsured, and this legislative provision permitted access to coverage for many as a result.[69]

In addition to accessibility and coverage considerations, the ACA also addressed patient costs and quality of care provided. Given the fact that patient outcomes have ranked so low compared to other countries despite the highest per capita investments, quality and costs have certainly been poorly managed. The ACA addressed costs to patients through creating competitive marketplaces of health insurance exchanges where insurance companies will compete for increased population pools, thus driving down patient health insurance costs in the process. Other measures established by the ACA include reductions in Medicare reimbursement rate increases for providers. With

---

68   Zuckerman, 2012.
69   Shi, 2015.

this constraint, providers have been forced to address costs.[70] As a result, more streamlined care, bundled care opportunities, and elimination of unnecessary services are taking place in an effort to lower patient costs and healthcare expenditures.

Costs were also constrained by placing limits on the amount health insurance companies could spend on administrative costs. If these companies exceeded a percentage of the premium spent on these cost areas, then penalties and premium refunds would be provided. This forced insurance companies to be leaner in their approach to health insurance coverage. Likewise, in addition to the creation of a public website for Americans to access and view insurance plans available, the ACA required the development of a uniform coverage document so consumers could easily compare different health insurance plans. By reducing the complexities of plans, consumers were better able to make educated decisions about their coverage based on a variety of factors including cost, quality, and services.[71]

The market exchanges will naturally compete not only on costs but also on quality of services. Different tier levels reflect different levels of cost sharing by consumers as well as different levels of care services available. However, the ACA requires all health plans to meet specific criteria in order to participate in the health insurance exchanges. Specifically, all must provide specific prevention services and health screenings, and immunizations must be provided to consumers without any out-of-pocket costs. By requiring certain essential health benefits, the ACA sought to raise the bar on basic health insurance coverage while moving in a direction that advocated prevention and health promotion over the treatment of disease alone.[72]

---

70   Obamacarefacts.com, "Affordable Care Act Summary," n.d., http://obamacarefacts.com/affordable-careact-summary/.
71   Ibid.
72   Ibid.

Other Important Aspects of the ACA

Other policies similarly addressed quality of care issues in healthcare. The ACA established a Patient Centered Outcome Research Institute, which examines outcomes for quality practice guidance, rate adjustment determinations, and other related policies to encourage higher quality care. Evidence-based practice is a focus of the institute since this has greater potential to provide better quality and lower cost services and higher value. Also, the ACA through the Centers for Medicare and Medicaid Innovations has supported the testing of new payment and delivery models of care through a variety of bundling options.[73] Those being identified as higher in quality outcomes and lower in cost will likely affect future healthcare policies.

While lack of access to healthcare and poor quality care result in preventable illness and death, these factors account for only 15 percent of such occurrences. Lack of education, behavioral choices, physical environments, and socioeconomic conditions account for 85 percent of factors that affect morbidity and mortality. With this in mind, key components of the ACA addressed some public health and population-based needs. Specifically, one of the goals of the ACA strives for general population health improvement. The IRS under the ACA requires all nonprofit hospitals to complete community health needs assessments every three years and to identify efforts being pursued to meet these needs. This offers new opportunities for hospitals and public health agencies to collaborate on population needs. In addition, a Prevention and Public Health Fund has been created by the ACA to invest in education, in public health efforts, and in community transformation grants.

In addition to these developments, the ACA addressed other areas of healthcare reform as well. In terms of Medicaid, the ACA maintained children's access to healthcare through CHIP programs while

---

73   Ibid.

simplifying the enrollment process. For older adults, the ACA also eliminated copays for routine preventive services charged by health insurance companies. Policies were also adopted that promote greater access to nutritional information for consumers. And community health center funding was enhanced to better serve public health measures at community levels.[74] While the ACA is often viewed through mandates and healthcare insurance exchanges, the legislation is much broader in scope when it comes to healthcare reform.

One of the important areas the ACA addresses involves long-term care for Americans. With the aging of the population and the rising prevalence of chronic disease, the expected demands for long-term care in the future are staggering. With this need in mind, the ACA adopted policies that support a number of areas related to long-term care. Specifically, the ACA supports expansion of home healthcare services in communities for older adults, and also requires greater consumer transparency among nursing homes in terms of their quality of care to enable better decision making and competition. The ACA also promotes the development of voluntary, self-funded programs through employers, which are funded through additional worker premium payments. The benefits of these programs can be used for long-term care services in the community and at home if a worker becomes disabled.[75]

The ACA also addressed the need for an increasing healthcare workforce for the future. Given the rising demand for healthcare services, workforce needs have been identified as a priority. The legislation supports state programs that establish scholarships, and loan forgiveness for professionals choosing to enter healthcare fields. This is particularly important for primary care services as well as allied health professional fields since a large burden of care will be for older adults in the community. While specific requirements are

---

74   Ibid.
75   Ibid.

not provided within the ACA, the support provided indicates this will be an ongoing concern for healthcare in general.[76]

One of the most notable aspects of the ACA in terms of reduced healthcare expenditures has been the reduction of overpayments and fraudulent claims. Specifically, the ACA actively has sought to eliminate overpayments to providers and health insurance companies, as these represent a significant portion of healthcare expenditures that could be quickly remedied. Likewise, the ACA also supports state sanctions and restrictions for providers and companies that participate in fraudulent reimbursement activities, encouraging interstate cooperation to limit such behaviors in the future. As a result of these efforts, the ACA has saved millions of dollars in healthcare expenditures in a short time.[77]

Last, the ACA has also sought to address rising pharmaceutical costs. Though restriction of innovation and advancing technologies is not a desirable pursuit, the need to provide affordable medications to Americans is certainly important. As a result, the ACA supports the extension of pharmaceutical programs that offer medication discounts for low-income consumers. It also promotes greater development of generic medications among pharmaceutical companies while reducing competitive pressures between generic drugs and brand-name drugs.[78] This will continue to be an important area of cost savings for Americans in the future, especially as chronic disease prevalence rises.

Criticisms of the ACA

As previously noted, one of the most controversial aspects of the ACA was the required individual mandate and the development of

---

76   Ibid.
77   Ibid.
78   Ibid.

healthcare exchanges by states. Because consumer access was largely addressed through Medicaid expansion, and because states experience substantial costs related to Medicaid programs regardless, many states resisted the changes. Politically conservatives states particularly pushed back against ACA legislation, claiming federal legislation interfered with state rights too significantly. The costs states would experience in developing health insurance exchanges, their administration, as well as the subsequent costs related to Medicaid program expansion would place tremendous financial burdens on states.[79]

Understanding these economic concerns, the ACA did allow for the federal government to cover the costs of Medicaid expansion for states for the initial three years after its initiation. However, after this, states would have increasing responsibilities in sharing the costs associated with Medicaid expansion. In addition, the ACA threatened to withhold all federal funding for states related to Medicaid should they choose not to adopt the requirements listed in the ACA. This was a significant concern for any state since federal funding for existing Medicaid program support is essential for financial viability. As a result, many states decided to fight back against these policies.[80]

Overall, twenty-eight states decided to file suit against the US government based on a perception that the ACA was unconstitutional. First, these states claimed the ACA violated the constitutional rights of individuals by imposing a penalty on individuals (through the individual mandate tax penalty) who choose not to participate in health insurance programs. Proponents of the ACA stated the Commerce Clause of the US Constitution permits the federal government to tax for revenues when an issue concerns the general welfare of everyone in the nation. However, opponents of the ACA claimed that

79 Sarah Horton, Cesar Abadía, Jessica Mulligan, and Jennifer Jo Thompson, "Critical Anthropology of Global Health 'Takes a Stand' Statement: A Critical Medical Anthropological Approach to the US's Affordable Care Act," *Medical Anthropology Quarterly* 28, no. 1 (2014): 1–22.
80 Ibid.

the Commerce Clause was not intended to be used for noneconomic activity but for economic actions only. In this case, failure of an individual to spend money on healthcare results in taxation penalties, which is novel. This debate was substantial enough that the case went before the Supreme Court in 2012, and the court ruled in favor of the ACA's constitutionality on this issue by a vote of 5–4.[81]

While the ACA and the federal government won the battle over the individual mandate, the second issue upon which the court ruled was less favorable. When it came to restricting Medicaid funding to states based on their nonparticipation in ACA programs, the Supreme Court ruled that such actions represented excessive centralized government power, and states should not be threatened with federal withholding of complete Medicaid funding when existing Medicaid programs remained in place. This was a notable win for many states, and to date, more than two dozen states have continued to resist participation in health insurance exchanges and Medicaid expansion. Though this figure gradually declines each year, the result has been to dilute the potential beneficial effects on patient access to health insurance in these states.[82]

In addition to these legal battles, many other criticisms of the ACA exist as well. The overall ACA programs were modeled from recent health insurance legislations in the state of Massachusetts. While access to healthcare was enhanced in Massachusetts and healthcare costs reduced, the state program also experienced increases in administrative and bureaucratic costs. Therefore, one of the criticisms of the ACA relates to an increased need for clerical and midlevel professional staff associated with ACA programs and their implementation. Likewise, by nature of the ACA requirements, individuals are now faced with increased complexities concerning health insurance coverage. While uniform documents and health insurance exchanges make

---

81　Klein, 2012.
82　Horton, 2014.

it easier to compare insurance plans, issues related to government subsidies, different tier levels of insurance, and individual mandate penalty taxes place greater demands on consumers.[83]

The ACA also fails to adequately address many other areas of healthcare. Specifically, dental, vision, and mental health coverage is lacking under ACA programs, and these reflect chronic areas where Americans lack healthcare coverage. These areas as well as complementary and alternative medical therapies are typically excluded from many insurance plans or significantly undersupported. As a result, consumers must pay significant out-of-pocket costs for these aspects of healthcare, or they neglect them altogether. Overall healthcare costs continue to be high for individuals in these areas as a result, and this serves to undermine the overall benefits of the ACA in relation to costs, access, and quality of care.[84]

Specific groups have clearly benefitted from ACA policies, For example, women who were previously charged higher insurance premiums or excluded from insurance plans now have access to equal coverage. In addition, women also now receive contraception coverage as part of ACA plan requirements. Similarly, patients with HIV and AIDS can no longer be refused insurance coverage either. However, health insurance coverage for undocumented individuals in the country has not been addressed, and this segment of the population does contribute to healthcare expenditures overall. While undocumented individuals as well as prisoners, the impoverished, and certain ethnic and religious groups are exempt from the individual mandate provisions of the ACA, access and costs for these groups are poorly considered under current ACA programs.[85]

In relation to hospitals, the ACA eliminated disproportionate share funding to those facilities that primarily served low-income

---

83   Ibid.
84   Ibid.
85   Ibid.

populations. Previously, additional Medicaid funds were available to these hospitals, but this was eliminated with the Medicaid expansion programs of the ACA. Thus, in states that have failed to adopt ACA Medicaid expansion, such hospitals face not only reduced incomes from this policy change, but they also fail to benefit from the addition of newly insured patients related to this expansion. Concerns exist that these hospitals will react to these situations by charging indigent individuals higher fees or by excluding undocumented individuals from their community health programs. As a result, this could lead to an increase in healthcare disparities rather than a reduction.[86]

The strongest criticisms regarding the ACA have come from conservative political groups. Philosophical differences account for many of these criticisms, and as a result, new proposals to address healthcare reform have been made. One of the most recent proposals is a comprehensive healthcare reform encompassing numerous pieces of legislation as well as the repeal of Obamacare. Speaker of the House Paul Ryan has detailed these reform changes with specific criticisms of the ACA that include a lack of provider choice, the presence of a highly regulated system, and an increase in costs rather than the opposite. In addition, opponents have made criticisms related to a decline in quality of care, stating that using a Medicaid system to support millions of Americans is contrary to high level of care.[87]

Alternative proposed plans seek to similarly encourage transparency and innovation while also encouraging portability of coverage and provider choice. Specific programs that would seek to accomplish this would include health savings accounts (HSAs), which would be used in tandem to support high-deductible health plans. In addition, private health plans would be allowed to move with individuals from employer to employer, and small business pools would be created to

---

86   Ibid.
87   Office of Speaker of the House, "A better way: Our vision for a confident America," 2016, https://abetterway.speaker.gov/_assets/pdf/ABetterWay-HealthCare-PolicyPaper.pdf.

assist these businesses in providing employee-based coverage. Other measures also include the ability to reward employees for wellness behaviors, options for continued employer self-insured programs, and medical tort reform to reduce risks and the practice of defensive medicine. Through these programs, access would reportedly be improved, and costs would be reduced.[88]

As part of these alternative proposals, patient protections would be included. The ability to cancel or drop someone from health insurance coverage would be prohibited on the basis of preexisting conditions, and lifetime limits would also not be allowed. And, like the ACA, individuals under age twenty-six years could be included on parental health plans. But other notable changes would be present. These include the inability to use tax dollars for abortion services, and a complete reform of Medicaid programs while preserving Medicare itself. Likewise, high-risk patient pools would be created, along with state innovation grants to assist states with rising healthcare coverage costs. Last, limits on tax credits for employers would be created to reduce the overall magnitude of government subsidies. These proposals suggest lower costs and a higher quality of healthcare will result.[89] But while this reflects an alternative approach, the proof such directions would prove more effective than ACA remains to be validated.

Without question, the ACA has led to increased access to coverage and care for many individuals. As of 2016, over eleven million people had signed up for health insurance programs using health insurance exchanges. However, this figure was expected to be significantly higher, with some projections doubling this figure. In addition, some counties in states where health insurance exchanges exist have only one insurance provider. Roughly 7 percent of the population resides in such counties. Though the uninsured rate has dropped to 9 percent, the rates for the underinsured have not fallen as much. By definition,

---

88   Ibid.
89   Ibid.

the underinsured reflect individuals who spend more than 10 percent of their income on out-of-pocket expenses. With higher premiums, copays, and deductibles, this specific segment of the population has not declined as dramatically under current ACA provisions.[90]

Finally, provider participation remains a concern under current ACA programs with specific concerns over Medicaid enrollees. Statistics have shown that only slightly more than half of all physician providers are accepting new Medicaid patients, and only slightly more than three-quarters accept new Medicare patients. Low reimbursement rates have encouraged some providers to exclude this population segment from their practice. Therefore, the ACA has created a situation where increased access to coverage is associated with reduced provider options and potentially lower quality of care. Despite expanding Medicaid coverage to accommodate more people, some suggest the programs serve to perpetuate inequality in healthcare services.[91]

Overall, the ACA has accomplished many positive goals in terms of reforming healthcare policies. The program has eliminated limits on coverage, exclusions based on preexisting conditions, and coverage denials. Likewise, the ACA placed limits on what insurance companies could spend in administrative costs, and a minimum standard of benefits was defined that all insurance plans had to provide. However, at the same time, ACA made many concessions. Negotiations with private insurers resulted in a lack of consideration for a single payer system or for a public health insurance option. And options to lower prescription drug prices for Medicare patients through negotiations with pharmaceutical companies were avoided. Because of this, the ACA can be seen as a major piece of legislative reform that addressed

90   Carolyn Y. Johnson, "Healthcare Exchange Sign-ups Fall Far Short of Forecasts," *Washington Post*, 2016, https://www.washingtonpost.com/business/economy/health-care-exchange-sign-ups-fall-far-short-of-forecasts/2016/08/27/3d93f602-6895-11e6-99bf-f0cf3a6449a6_story.html?utm_term=.baa5b5021a0b.
91   Horton, 2014.

many problems of the healthcare system, but at the same time, it also left many issues unattended or inadequately managed.[92]

Shifting Healthcare Dynamics for the Twenty-First Century

Given the prior descriptions regarding today's healthcare, a number of current challenges exist in striving to attain an effective, quality-focused system. The one that receives the most attention is naturally the rising costs of healthcare, since this figure is roughly 17 percent of our nation's gross domestic product. Healthcare expenditures rose dramatically in the 1970s and 1980s, somewhat stabilized in the 1990s, and then rose again during the early part of this century. And despite attempts to contain costs through different payment structures and through the use of technologies, minimal gains have been made. The cost of healthcare is by far the most pressing challenge, as many experts believe the current trends are unsustainable. This is particularly true given the aging of the population and the rise in prevalence of those with chronic illnesses.

Another major challenge relates to the issue of quality. In order to assess healthcare quality, it must first be defined. According to the Institute of Medicine, quality services are those that result in the desired outcome based on current medical knowledge. According to the Agency for Healthcare Research and Quality, quality care is delivering the right services at the right time to the right person in the right way so optimal results are attained. Even with these definitions, however, some ambiguity exists. For example, a provider may consider high quality as a depth of knowledge about a patient's condition while ignoring the costs involved to acquire that knowledge. A consumer may perceive quality based on the actual delivery system in terms of wait times, inconveniences, as well as health results. And insurers may perceive quality as measures that reduce risk while also

---

92   Ibid.

controlling costs. Depending on who determines quality measures affects whether quality is or is not perceived.

While policies are beginning to change concerning quality measures, recent abilities to assess quality have been difficult. For one thing, because treatment recommendations vary somewhat among providers, determining optimal quality results can be challenging if a preferred treatment is not defined. Likewise, providers who perform higher quality care have not necessarily been rewarded, and those performing poor care have not been penalized. In fact, some poor quality care providers might even be rewarded, as is the case with those who perform excessive services. In order to address quality in healthcare, some ability to define quality based on value must be determined, and incentives must be in place to encourage higher quality care.

The patient-physician relationship has always represented the central focus of all healthcare activities. Since the beginning of organized healthcare, this relationship has been viewed as sacred, private, and essential to effective health services. However, over the past century, dozens of other healthcare professionals and stakeholders have been included in these services and care. Currently, for each physician in the US, ten healthcare administrators exist. Consumer access to healthcare is meticulously regulated and designed to presumably facilitate this access and to monitor the efficiency of the whole system. Unfortunately, for one reason or the other, this efficiency has not been very effective, and patient-physician interactions have become less robust.[93]

Over this same period of time, care services that have not been adequately reimbursed have declined in number. For example, home visits by physicians are almost nonexistent, and the time taken to inquire about specific stresses, home environments, and family dynamics has

---

93   Heather Kathryn Ross, "The Great Healthcare Bloat: 10 Administrators for Every 1 US Doctor," *Healthline.com*, 2013, http://www.healthline.com/health-news/policy-ten-administrators-for-every-one-us-doctor-092813.

diminished. The *Marcus Welby, M.D.* model of practicing medicine has essentially become extinct and replaced by something completely different. This new model, which focuses on efficiency, volume, and documentation, has resulted in total dissatisfaction for both patients and physicians alike. But hope for change exists. Advances in communications and computer technologies provide a pivotal and transformative opportunity in healthcare that, if properly appreciated by all parties, can reestablish the value of the patient-physician relationship and enhance healthcare at the same time.

As previously noted, consumers will accept almost any type of care they can easily access. Other healthcare stakeholders work behind the scenes to qualify and regulate care for the consumer with the goal of maximizing access and quality. Unfortunately, early twentieth-century healthcare hindered access to some forms of healthcare for the uninsured. This resulted in subsequent legislation to try to improve healthcare services for this population. In 1986, the Emergency Medical Treatment and Active Labor Act (EMTALA) was passed, which required hospital emergency rooms that accepted Medicare payments to provide appropriate care services to all populations presenting for treatment. Emergency rooms had to provide care, regardless of whether these individuals were able to pay or were legal citizens. And if the facility considered a transfer, the patient's condition had to be stabilized. In other words, one facility could not "dump" this population on other facilities to avoid the regulations.[94]

Certainly this legislation allowed greater access to care services for the uninsured, but at the same time, this legislation undermined quality of care in several ways. First, the legislation failed to account for any form of reimbursement for the facilities that provided care to these individuals. Therefore, the legislation resulted in significant financial pressures on these institutions and led to a rise in medical

---

94   American College of Emergency Physicians, "EMTALA," 2016, https://www.acep.org/news-media-top-banner/emtala/.

bankruptcies for patients. In addition, the uninsured would often avoid routine care and health screenings since access to these services was not expanded. Instead, uninsured people would wait until a medical condition was urgent or emergent, and then they would seek care through emergency rooms. Not only did this result in higher costs of care and an inappropriate use of healthcare resources, but it also reduced quality of care, patient outcomes, and quality of life.

With the passage of the ACA and Obamacare, the expectation was that the volume of uninsured patients, as well as all patients, would decline as a result of higher insured percentages and better routine care services. However, a 2015 poll released by the American College of Emergency Physicians found that a majority of emergency room physicians reported an increase in patient volumes. Certainly this is counterintuitive to expected results, but some suggest the shortage of primary care services failed to meet patient demand even as heightened access occurred. As a result, uninsured as well as some insured patients still utilized high-cost resources in emergency departments for their medical care.[95]

In considering these phenomena, incentives and reimbursement strategies must be considered when developing new regulations and legislation to enhance access to consumer healthcare. In an effort to address the increase in chronic disease care management, access to healthcare services needs to be made available to all citizens. But at the same time, providers and physicians must be encouraged to manage this increased patient load. Tax incentives for physicians could be one type of strategy to encourage participation. Another possible strategy could be tax exemption for providers who offer care to Medicaid patients and other groups, similar to provisions offered nonprofit hospitals. Whatever the strategy, neglecting incentive

---

95   Laura Ungar and Jayne O'Donnell, "Contrary to goals, ER visits rise under Obamacare," *USA Today*, May 4, 2015, http://www.usatoday.com/story/news/nation/2015/05/04/emergency-room-visits-rise-under-affordable-care-act/26625571/.

reimbursement altogether has been shown to result in failed outcomes and objectives thus far.

The increase in chronic disease requires a shift in strategies and approaches to access healthcare services. While encouraging centers of excellence for stroke, trauma, spine injuries, and cardiovascular conditions in hospitals has some inherent advantages, the same approach for hypertension, diabetes, and obesity in outpatient centers will not be as effective. The statistics demonstrate the need for a new approach. Nearly two hundred million individuals in the US had at least one chronic disease last year, and seventy-five million had two or more. Direct costs of care for this population has been estimated at $75 million, with indirect costs adding another $800 million. Prevention services, health promotion, and enhanced routine care is needed for this population to reduce these costs and to enhance overall quality of care.[96]

Utilizing emergency rooms as sources of primary care health services is not the answer. Overall, about 12 percent of all emergency room visits require hospital admission. The remaining patients are most often referred back to their primary care providers. However, the coordination of care between the emergency room and the primary care provider is often haphazard. In addition, hospitalists, a position that has grown in most hospitals throughout the nation, often manage these same patients in the emergency room and hospital setting.[97] Yet, their approach to care is more focused on acute management rather than long-term care. Thus, both emergency room and hospitalist care fails to provide the optimal services needed for patients suffering with chronic diseases.

One of the key lessons learned from Obamacare is that a segment of the population will continue not to seek healthcare insurance coverage

96 Centers for Disease Control (CDC), "Chronic Disease Overview," 2016, https://www.cdc.gov/chronicdisease/overview/.

97 Centers for Disease Control (CDC), "Emergency Department Visits," 2016, https://www.cdc.gov/nchs/fastats/emergency-department.htm.

but will instead accept tax penalties. Therefore, access to healthcare should not be solely aligned with whether or not an individual has health insurance coverage or not. Because of this fact, some level of access should be provided to all individuals regardless of whether health insurance is in place. In addition, processes should be put into place to identify people with complex conditions and high socioeconomic risk factors for poor health. Once identified, additional services should be made available to reduce utilization of high-cost resources and promote better long-term health. Insurance providers should explore new ways to offer new products and services to such markets through the use of advanced technologies. These approaches offer a more logical approach to healthcare in comparison to strategies pursued so far.

Recent financial analyses examining healthcare spending from 1996 to 2013 have demonstrated that healthcare spending grew 3.5 percent per year during that time. In addition, out of 155 diseases, twenty of these conditions accounted for more than half of all the spending. While diabetes mellitus led the list, this condition in addition to heart disease, low back pain, hypertension, and fall-related injuries accounted for nearly 20 percent of healthcare spending, resulting in $437 billion spent in 2013 alone.[98] Addressing such areas of healthcare spending is imperative for the future.

New challenges exist for the twenty-first century in regard to healthcare. Consumers in particular have heightened expectations in many areas, which affects a variety of healthcare stakeholders. With advances in HITs, patients assume healthcare reports will be available almost instantaneously, and likewise, they expect their providers to have immediate access to diagnostic reports and results. In addition, access to numerous health websites and applications has resulted in a

---

98   Joseph L. Dieleman, Ranju Baral, Maxwell Birger, Anthony L. Bui, Anne Bulchis, Abigail Chapin, Hannah Hamavid, et al., "US Spending on Personal Health Care and Public Health, 1996–2013," *JAMA* 316, no. 24 (Dec. 27, 2016): 2627–2646.

more educated healthcare consumer. Not only is information readily available, but patients can self-interpret test results, symptom data, and other information, which can create anxiety on the one hand and greater discernment of healthcare services on the other. All of these changes serve to place greater pressure on physicians and providers in answering patient questions and in providing more efficient and qualitative services.

Recent surveys have demonstrated these shifts in healthcare toward a more consumer-oriented model. Specifically, patients have indicated heightened interest in being able to understand their diagnosis, own their own medical records, and enjoy total access to reports and chart notes. In other words, consumers want to play a more active and engaged role in their own healthcare. Physicians, on the other hand, have expressed a degree of uneasiness associated with technological advances and with changing levels of information access and engagement with patients. Overall, most younger physicians describe reluctance to allow patients access to their complete medical records, and generally, twice as many patients felt they should have immediate access to lab results before physician review when compared to physicians. In fact, 70 percent of physicians felt lab results should be physician-reviewed prior to being released to patients. Notably, these opinions are affected by different views of the healthcare process, levels of physician maturity, and perceived risks involved.[99]

Medical record ownership reflects another area where different views between patients and physicians exist. Among physicians, roughly 50 percent believe the medical record should be owned by the patient while the other half believes the opposite. In contrast, the vast majority of patients feel medical records belong to patients

---

99   Debra L. Boeldt, Nathan E. Wineinger, Jill Waalen, Shreya Gollamudi, Adam Grossberg, Steven R. Steinhubl, Anna McCollister-Slipp, Marc A. Rogers, Carey Silvers, and Eric J. Topol, "How Consumers and Physicians View New Medical Technology: Comparative Survey," *Journal of Medical Internet Research* 17, no. 9 (2015): e215.

themselves. Since these issues are often regulated by state laws, this might be a source of resolution, but extremely few states presently address this issue. Among the ones that do, both sides have been supported in different states. As patient involvement and engagement increase, and as healthcare shifts to a more patient-centric model, this issue will be an important one to address.[100]

When it comes to the use of email or video technologies to manage chronic diseases and provide medication prescriptions, patients and physicians also differ greatly. In fact, twice as many patients as physicians acknowledge an adequate level of comfort in these areas using these HITs. Patients tend on average to have less concern about privacy and a greater desire to utilize new technologies for greater efficiency and convenience. Even so, a significant number of both groups expressed concerns regarding remote treatment options. Healthcare data security breaches have increased significantly in the last two years, Overall, nearly 90 percent of healthcare organizations admit some type of security breach in this area during this time period, and costs associated with these breaches are in the millions of dollars.[101]

Having identified chronic disease care as a priority for the twenty-first century, the use of HIT to address better access to care in this area offers strong potential. With a reduction in the number of uninsured individuals and a rise in chronic disease prevalence, technology can provide a means by which primary care shortages and limited access to chronic disease care can be counterbalanced. As greater pressures develop to shift from volume-based care to value-based care, different mentalities must be considered. Likewise, attending to ambulatory care, at-home care, and continuity of care, new approaches must be developed. And at the same time, physicians must be included and be active participants in the process. Failing to do so can have disastrous results in attaining the goals outlined for better

---

100   Ibid.
101   Ibid.

healthcare in the future. With this in mind, technologies that address physician concerns and provide desired services will likely offer the best overall outcomes moving forward.

While involving physicians in the use of technologies to enhance healthcare will be important in the twenty-first century, managing regulatory changes will similarly be important. Beginning in 2017, physicians will begin submitting specific data requirements to CMS so physician performance can be assessed. Under the Medicare Access and CHIP Reauthorization Act of 2015 (MACRA), physicians will be assessed under the Merit-Based Incentive Payment System (MIPS) and the Advanced Alternative Payment Models (APMs). Based on four categories related to quality, meaningful use, practice improvement, and resource use, scores from 0 to 100 will be awarded each physician. Depending on the score, adjustments to Medicare reimbursements will be determined for that physician, which could result in increased, decreased, or no change in payments. While actual reimbursement changes will not take effect until 2019, performance scores will be determined beginning in 2017. This will require physicians who participate in Medicare Part B to shift their perspectives on patient care strategies and results.[102]

It is noteworthy that CMS does qualify physician encounters with patients under the MIPS program differently depending on the interaction type. Both patient-facing and non-patient-facing encounters will be considered, and each will affect payment adjustments as a result. Patient-facing encounters will naturally involve general office visits, surgical procedures, and other outpatient encounters where the patient appears for assessment in person. However, it will also apply to telehealth encounters under the MIPS program. It should also be

---

102   Richard J. Zall and Edward S. Kornreich, "The Future of Medicare Physician Reimbursement," *Law360*, May 13, 2016, http://www.proskauer.com/files/News/78231053-6cc3-4c6d-8296-f2084c0e3937/Presentation/NewsAttachment/7f3aa4cc-fbc0-4d85-bfc2-80cdd67e45dd/The%20Future%20Of%20Medicare%20Physician%20Reimbursement.pdf.

noted that payment adjustments increase over time with maximal adjustments, capping at 4 percent in 2019 and extending gradually up to 9 percent after 2022.[103]

The overall MIPS performance score will be based on four specific categories, and each of the categories will affect the weighted composite measure to different degrees since percent weights for each category vary over time. The first category involves quality of care, which requires six measures to be reported, including at least one outcome measure and one cost-cutting measure. Other measures can include data on patient safety, efficiency, patient experience, care coordination, or appropriate use. For the initial year in 2019, this measure will account for 50 percent of the total performance score.[104]

The second category is the advancement of care information. Related to information sharing and use, this category has been previously classified as meaningful use data, and it will comprise 25 percent of a physician's total performance score initially. Within this category physicians will report the use of various HITs in their practice with particular attention to health information exchange and interoperability. While barriers to these latter two areas exist and are beyond physician control in many instances, MIPS will force physicians to become more aware of these issues and advocate for positive change.[105]

Clinical practice improvement activities will represent the third category and account for 15 percent of the composite performance score. Notably, this category has the greatest degree of flexibility for physicians, as they are allowed to establish their own practice goals, and over ninety practice improvement activities are recognized by CMS. Examples of some common practice improvement activities might involve care coordination, patient safety enhancements, and

---

103   Ibid.
104   Ibid.
105   Ibid.

engagement with beneficiaries. A minimum number of activities is not required, but physicians are expected to be involved in such activities for at least ninety days annually.[106]

The fourth category involves the use of resources, and this category does not require physicians to be involved in a specific reporting measure. Instead, CMS will examine two specific measures internally related to a physician's Medicare billings. These will include total costs per capita for all Medicare beneficiaries as well as Medicare spending per beneficiary. Different measures will be examined within these areas for different physician specialties, and this category will account for 10 percent of a physician's performance score initially.[107] Naturally, these measures are more favorable when spending per capita is reduced for healthcare services.

While the primary focus of the MIPS performance scores will be to assess physician performance relevant to Medicare reimbursement adjustments, the MIPS program also is relevant to public transparency. The performance scores will eventually be available for public viewing for MIPS physicians, thus allowing consumers to choose physicians based on composite scores. Likewise, CMS plans to make quality and resource use scores readily available to physicians beginning in 2017 to provide feedback for change and to ensure accuracy in reporting. It should also be noted that a physician who believes errors or discrepancies exist can request a targeted review by CMS. However, additional appeals processes do not exist.[108]

In addition to the MIPS performance scoring measures, MACRA also defined APMs, or advanced alternative payment models. Example of an APM would be an accountable care organization (ACO) or a patient-centered medical home (PCMH). APMs represent clinician and clinical groups that pursue high-quality care in a highly

---

106   Ibid.
107   Ibid.
108   Ibid.

coordinated fashion. Specifically, APMs must require the use of EHR technologies, provide reimbursement healthcare services based on quality performance measures, and either be at-risk for significant levels of monetary loss or meet defining characteristics of a medical home under the Social Security Act.[109] As defined, it is evident the goal is to incentivize quality, value, and efficiency while reducing overall costs.

If physicians meet these requirements for an APM, they may be exempt from reporting performance measures and have the potential for additional financial bonuses. However, the percent of time and income under these APMs will progressively increase for physicians in order to realize these benefits. Currently, physicians involved in an APM must meet financial risk criteria which can include the withholding of a payment, reduction in reimbursement rates, or a requirement to pay back CMS if spending exceeded expected levels. The total risk for the APM must also be at least 4 percent of the overall spending projections for the APM.[110]

Initially, only patients that fall within Medicare services will be included within the determination of whether or not a physician can be considered part of an APM. However, in time, other patients can also be included. In 2021, CMS will include an all-payers option where other patients in APMs will be included in determining whether or not a physician meets criteria for an APM. The same criteria as previously noted will be required for these patient care services in making this determination, but it will expand consideration for the inclusion of additional physicians who may not meet the guidelines for Medicare patients alone.[111]

In essence, MIPS and APMs reflect a flexible system where physicians can move from one quality care program to another. All

---

109   Ibid.
110   Ibid.
111   Ibid.

physicians involved in an APM are considered MIPS-eligible physicians and will be subjected to performance reporting. Over time, the expectation is that an increasing number of physicians will be involved in APMs based on the reduced reporting requirements and financial incentives present. If adequate participation in Medicare Part B exists, physicians will be required to participate in MIPS and provide reporting data so that performance scores can be determined, reimbursement rates adjusted, and public transparency measures pursued. But if a physician participates in an APM to an adequate degree, reporting requirements and reimbursement adjustments may be avoided since risk is being shared already through the APM. Given this scenario, growth of APMs is expected.[112]

Healthcare in the twenty-first century poses many opportunities as well as challenges for physicians. Current regulatory changes, including Obamacare, have taught the nation some valuable lessons, including those related to improving patient access to care services. While access was enhanced under this legislation for many, high numbers of patients continued to utilize high cost centers of care while neglecting prevention and health-promotion activities. Physician shortages and lack of physician involvement reflect two key areas which were overlooked in this process.

Currently, regulatory shifts are moving in a different direction. Reimbursement penalties and incentives are being aligned with quality of care outcomes, healthcare spending measures, and resource utilization. Likewise, the meaningful use of technologies is being encouraged, as is risk-sharing activities by physicians. This is all occurring in an environment where heightened transparency and accountability is being promoted, and in a setting where consumers have progressively higher expectations of service, engagement, and

---

112   Ibid.

participation. These summarize the key areas of importance for physicians as they seek to best navigate twenty-first-century healthcare.

Naturally, change is difficult and tends to provoke anxiety, but at the same time, change invites a chance to adopt better measures of care. In relation to twenty-first-century healthcare, these opportunities certainly exist, and at the same time, they allow a chance for physicians to pursue stronger physician-patient relations. This remains the foundation of healthcare services and adopting new methods of care, which strengthens this foundation while enhancing value, quality, and efficiency result in win-win scenarios for all healthcare stakeholders.

CHAPTER 3

Twenty-First-Century Healthcare Informatics

What Is Healthcare Informatics?

Over the course of the last several decades, information technologies have advanced at a tremendous pace. Nearly every sector has experienced a technological shift as a result, and healthcare is not different. While healthcare may lag behind other industries in utilizing information and communication technologies (ICT) to their full extent, changes have occurred regardless. And the area that deals with these types of changes is termed healthcare informatics.

Healthcare informatics encompasses a broad spectrum of activities. In essence, healthcare informatics reflects a multidisciplinary field that combines information science, computer science, and various health sciences in an effort to advance healthcare services. These advances seek to improve the quality, efficiency, effectiveness, and accessibility of healthcare services in the process, and involve the ongoing analysis, development, implementation, and evaluation of ICT systems. Through the use of data and information, various areas of healthcare can be enhanced. As a result, resource utilization is improved, better guidelines developed, and an array of ICT tools allow better healthcare outcomes.

While ICT in healthcare is a rather broad field, clinical informatics deals with direct patient care as it pertains to information and data. ICT systems seek better patient safety and outcomes while promoting patient-centered care and overall effectiveness. Specialists with expertise in this particular area are termed clinical informatics specialists, and this appears to be an advancing area of expertise in healthcare informatics overall. In fact, a physician-only certification process in clinical informatics was launched in 2013 sponsored by the American Board of Preventive Medicine. Qualifying physicians who complete an approved twenty-four-month fellowship in clinical informatics are eligible to take the certification exam. Based on the number of physicians pursuing this certification, this clearly is an up and coming area of interest.[113]

Clinical informatics specialists can have an array of responsibilities and duties. Assessing ICT needs in clinical arenas are common tasks, as are the procurement, development, implementation, and management of clinical information systems. From electronic health records to clinical decision support systems to larger data analytics systems, these specialists facilitate better healthcare outcomes through the use of ICT. And given the need for enhanced quality and safety of care at lower cost and resource utilization, these experts will undoubtedly serve an increasing role in the healthcare environment as the future unfolds.

The role of healthcare informatics occupies a significant component of healthcare activities even today. Combining information and computer sciences with health sciences has created opportunities as well as new challenges. The potential for enhanced efficiency, quality, and efficacy of patient care exists, but at the same time we should be aware of various pitfalls and areas of concern. The following sections will cover the history of healthcare informatics in addition to some of the key opportunities and challenges that exist with its use in healthcare.

113   "Clinical Informatics 2014 Diplomats," American Board of Preventive Medicine, December 2013.

History of Healthcare Informatics

Like most computer science fields, the role of informatics in healthcare began in the middle of the twentieth century. Sponsored by entities like the US Air Force and the National Institutes of Health (NIH), funding supported research and investigations in health-related fields beginning in the 1950s. After realizing the potential that computer technologies had in improving medical decision making, progressive investments then followed in subsequent decades. Millions of dollars were invested into the use of computers in various areas of biology and medicine, and a number of biomedical research centers began utilizing these tools and systems.[114]

Progress was initially made utilizing computer technologies both in clinical and research related fields. Computers enabled researchers to manage larger sample sizes of research participants, and they could perform more detailed data analytics as well. In addition, medical research databases and catalogs emerged, allowing greater access to healthcare information. And specific areas of interest, such as prosthetic development, benefitted from computer analyses of human movement through computer assistance. These advantages began to emerge during the 1960s and 1970s, and from this point, the integration of computer sciences and healthcare accelerated greatly.[115]

By the time the 1980s arrived, a number of organizations were investing heavily in the use of computer technologies in healthcare, including public entities such as the NIH and the Veterans Administration system, as well as larger private institutions like Massachusetts General Hospital and Kaiser Permanente. They introduced computer programming languages specific to clinical areas of interest, as well as the development of new clinical databases. Likewise, further

---

114   Dee McGonigle and Kathleen Mastrian, *Nursing Informatics and the Foundation of Knowledge*, Jones & Bartlett Publishers, 2014.
115   Ibid.

technological advances, such as graphic user interfaces, enabled the development of electronic health records (EHRs). Though these were rarely utilized in clinical practice at this point, the potential for their future use was already clear by this point in time. As a result, many private organizations began developing EHR and clinical practice management technologies.[116]

Despite the adoption of computer systems in other industries, healthcare was slow to adopt such technologies. Practice management systems were adopted earlier, with many healthcare facilities and organizations beginning to utilize these tools in the 1990s. However, EHR system use was much slower to catch on. Costs related to their purchase, a lack of interoperability and information sharing, and limitations in converting traditional clinical documentation to electronic documentation were all initial challenges. Not until the early part of the twenty-first century did such systems gain favor. This occurred not only because of technological advancements but also as a result of legislative incentives such as those outlined in the Health Information Technology for Economic and Clinical Health (HITECH) Act.

Today, the use of clinical information systems as well as other computer technologies is quite common in healthcare. Diagnosis and management activities, decision support systems, patient scheduling, medical billing, and a host of many other healthcare activities now utilize computing technologies and informatics. Technology use has led to reductions in medical errors, enhanced patient safety, development of evidence-based guidelines of care, and better efficiency of information sharing. But while computers have become common, clinical information systems continue to have problematic areas of concern. Thus, continued improvement in these systems remains a focus for the immediate future. Some of these challenges and areas for improvement will be covered in order to better grasp the current state of affairs.

116　Ibid.

Privacy and Cybersecurity Challenges

Today's healthcare industry is not as resilient to cyber intrusions when compared to the financial and retail sectors. A major hurdle arises from overseeing compliance with health data privacy regulations and efficiently handling the immense data flow among various work stations. Data loss and identity theft represent additional challenges. And lacking uniformity in how data is handled and shared adds another problematic dimension to a complex issue. A robust, cost effective, secure, and compliant foundation is thus an essential requirement for twenty-first-century healthcare.

Personally Identifiable Information (PII) and Patient Health Information (PHI) are increasingly being used and are governed by a number of complex policies that restrain access, audits, and the free-flow of big data. The legislative goals are to prevent unwarranted access by both authorized and nonauthorized users, to comply with audit requirements, and to link data sets among various networks and public Internet portals. In fact, the United States, Canada, Australia, and Europe share similar legislative initiatives to safeguard PII and PHI.

Healthcare is one of sixteen critical infrastructures that fall under Presidential Executive Order 13636 and its accompanying guideline "Framework for Improving Critical Infrastructure Cybersecurity" issued by the National Institute of Standards and Technology (NIST). While the use of the framework is currently voluntary, it provides a reasonable roadmap for best practices for cybersecurity policies and procedures.[117]

---

117   Lawrence A. Gordon, Martin P. Loeb, William Lucyshyn, and Lei Zhou, "Increasing Cybersecurity Investments in Private Sector Firms," *Journal of Cybersecurity* 1, no. 1 (2015): 3–17.

Threading the Data Integration Needle

Flexible data integration involves five specific phases. These include assessment, gap analysis, solution development, implementation, and steady-state maintenance. But these phases must be considered within the scope of cybersecurity. Despite these challenges, implementing measures for cyber-privacy and cybersecurity would add overall strength to the fabric of healthcare IT. One widely adopted model in cyber-privacy is to minimize the amount PII data overall. Audits would help limit its use to situations where a specific purpose is defined or when it is deemed necessary. Cybersecurity protocols identify, detect, protect, and respond to potential threats with the inherent agility to recover after an attack. Documenting where and why data is made available, and who has or had access to that data, adds another hurdle to successful and seamless data integration.[118]

Health organizations are major catalysts for current efforts involving healthcare data integration. Vertical and horizontal integration within a single organization or across multiple organizations can be daunting, and at times teetering on the edge of impossibility. Given these difficulties, initial assessment suggests that the user should be the focal point for any successful strategy related to data integration. The data is owned by the user, and it's easier for the data to chase its owner than the user to chase their own data. This is likely to continue to be a key strategy involving data integration.

Multiple healthcare platforms pose a challenge in narrowing the gap of data processing and integration across varying platforms. We propose that interoperability efforts for the twenty-first century include agile and provider-scalable mini platforms that would fit and move freely on a unisource ocean of patient data points devoid of PII. This approach, in our opinion, will better align patient and provider needs for the twenty-first century and will create a demand-driven consumer model.

---

118   Ibid.

Translational Science

The National Institutes of Health (NIH) established the National Center for Advancing Translational Sciences (NCATS) to facilitate fast and efficient delivery of new treatments and cures for disease discovered in the research environment. In addition, the one-size-fits-all model in healthcare is widely criticized by various stakeholders, and it appears healthcare is on the cusp of an on-demand, individually tailored delivery of healthcare. These pressures demand solutions, and clinicians are well positioned to address these issues in a direct and timely manner. Through these actions, providers will be more able to expand effective care plans and enhanced patient wellness.

Healthcare will be transformed by providing best-fit, real-time solutions that are widely available and cost effective. The art of medicine is based on evidence uncovered through observation and intuition. Clinicians can take advantage of the advances in computer technology and truly deliver personalized medicine with an emphasis on health rather than disease. By identifying the user as the primary point of care via portable and nonportable devices, other healthcare facilities then become secondary and tertiary points of care. This change conceptually offers great promise in enhancing how healthcare is delivered and its resultant effects on individual health outcomes.

Arbitrary Delivery of Care

The current model for the delivery of care outside the hospital can be called arbitrary at best. Delivery of care is triggered by either the patient or by the provider. Both can trigger delivery of care by scheduling an appointment. But these triggers may be premature, delayed, or even arbitrary at times. A patient can choose to delay care if symptoms are not overly concerning, or they may obtain premature care due to exaggerated subjective concerns which may or may not be objectively justifiable. At the same time, a provider may set up a return visit in an arbitrary fashion that lacks stratified standardized guidelines or falls short in aligning with the specific individual patient's problems.

In comparing these delivery of care models to other industries, clearly the healthcare care delivery system is significantly less efficient and effective. Let's take a look at OnStar, LLC as a prime example. OnStar is a subsidiary of General Motors (GM), which provides an array of automotive services to customers owning many models of GM vehicles. As an advanced IT company focused on safety, security, and mobility solutions, OnStar services over six million customers worldwide.

In the past, car owners struggled with a variety of issues, including locking one's keys in the car, car theft, unpredictable vehicle breakdowns, and several others. OnStar provided services to deal with such situations, such as automatic crash response, remote door unlock, GPS navigational tools, Wi-Fi provisions and 4G LTE services, and stolen vehicle assistance. In addition, OnStar coordinates with first responders when data from a crash predicts serious injury. In each case, data through an IT platform provides user-specific assistance.[119]

While these aspects of OnStar's service are exceptional, they also offer services involving up-to-date information about customers' vehicles. In addition to engine fluid levels, OnStar sends monthly diagnostic emails to consumers identifying specific areas of the car that may need attention. This information is also provided to dealers, who can anticipate and schedule service visits before a breakdown may occur. These are perfect examples of how IT and big data can provide health promotion and "disease prevention" for your car. Now imagine the same for the healthcare industry.

While the US healthcare system is a long way from an OnStar model, changes are moving in a favorable direction. In 2015, the Centers for

---

119   General Motors, "OnStar Creates Injury Severity Prediction to Improve Automatic Crash Response," May 20, 2009, http://media.gm.com/media/us/en/onstar/news.detail.html/content/Pages/news/us/en/2009/May/0520_OnStarPredictsInjury.html.

Medicare and Medicaid Services (CMS) approved reimbursement options for chronic care service provisions that included non-face-to-face care. While this type of care involves many parameters, a key component of this care relates to monitoring and surveillance of patients with chronic medical conditions before they experience an acute decline. Given the fact that chronic medical problems will soon represent nearly three-quarters of healthcare services, shifting incentives toward prevention services is important. Instead of waiting for a deterioration to occur, efforts to ensure proper care and the early detection of problems can greatly reduce costs while enhancing patient quality of life.

CMS lists the types of services it covers under chronic care management, and many of these involve healthcare informatics. Specifically, recording patient health information, developing an electronic care plan, and information sharing with care coordination are among key components of chronic care management. Advancing such programs through more advanced ICT solutions offers greater opportunities to enhance healthcare even further. As seen in the example that OnStar provides, greater focus on prevention and monitoring combined with advanced use of informatics could beneficially transform healthcare.

In this chapter, we have considered the current challenges as well as opportunities that exist in twenty-first-century healthcare. The advancement of healthcare informatics in recent decades, especially in clinical arenas, offers a tremendous chance to greatly improve the quality, efficiency, and efficacy of healthcare. But inherent challenges still exist which are unique to the healthcare sector. Fortunately, innovative solutions can tackle these problems and create a healthcare system conducive to better resource utilization and quality outcomes. And through these solutions, enhanced patient-provider relations can also occur further add value to the system.

CHAPTER 4

A Global Perspective on Health Needs and Challenges

When considering healthcare needs and issues, major challenges exist well beyond the borders of the United States. Worldwide health needs are astounding, and these become most notable in lower income, developing nations. But while these issues are disturbing, they do offer great opportunities for change and for new policies and approaches. The ability to utilize advancing technologies and interactive platforms to enhance access to healthcare services offers great hope. Such opportunities can make powerful impacts in every stage of healthcare, including screenings, prevention education, monitoring, and surveillance, as well as evaluations and therapies.

In order to best appreciate the opportunities such technologies may offer, we need a deeper understanding of worldwide health issues. The most significant worldwide health challenge today involves noncommunicable disease. Noncommunicable diseases differ from those which can be spread through various infectious routes in that they are often affected by lifestyle choices and environments and are thus preventable. In addition, most forms of noncommunicable diseases are chronic, and they impact healthcare systems and patient lives over an extended period of time, causing significant economic impact and resource depletion.

According to the World Health Organization (WHO), a total of fifty-six million deaths occurred in 2012. Of these deaths, thirty-eight million, or 68 percent, could be attributed to chronic diseases. Of these chronic disease deaths, an estimated 40 percent could have been prevented through changes in lifestyle, environments, and management.

And out of these deaths, roughly sixteen million affected individuals less than seventy years of age. These figures are staggering, but the expected growth of these numbers is even more concerning. The WHO projects that by the year 2030, the number of deaths per year from chronic disease will increase to fifty-two million. Because of population aging, increasing longevity, and specific epidemics such as obesity, chronic diseases will become more prevalent and result in higher mortality rates.[120]

Chronic diseases affect all nations in terms of healthcare expenditures and mortality. However, lower- to middle-income nations appear to be hit the hardest, suffering 75 percent of all chronic disease deaths, as well as 82 percent of all premature deaths. Chronic disease rates in these nations pose barriers to sustainable development and rises in per capita income levels.[121] Resources are constantly being depleted in the management of these conditions, resulting in a lack of funds for prevention and health promotion. As a result, such countries are constantly trying to catch up in a seemingly losing battle.

While the vast majority of countries have funds to support disease screenings, primary prevention efforts, health programs, and disease surveillance, nations throughout Africa and in the Eastern Mediterranean regions are among those with the lowest sources of funds. Of countries sampled by the WHO, 6 percent had no funding stream for such services. And among low income countries, this figure rose to 18 percent. In addition, the areas which were least well funded included disease surveillance, disease monitoring, healthcare capacity building, and rehabilitation services.[122] When funding is lacking for such programs, nations become unable to advance and progress.

Given these statistics, the WHO has a goal to reduce the prevalence of chronic diseases by 25 percent or more by 2025. Four major

---

120   World Health Organization (WHO), *Global Status Report on Non-Communicable Diseases 2014* (Switzerland: WHO Press, 2014).
121   Ibid.
122   Ibid.

areas of chronic disease have been identified as priority conditions based on the number of deaths associated with them annually. These conditions include cardiovascular disease, which caused 17.5 million deaths in 2012; cancer-related conditions, resulting in 21.7 million deaths; chronic respiratory conditions, causing four million deaths; and diabetes mellitus, which resulted in 1.5 million deaths.[123] Reducing the mortality and prevalence rates of these conditions will garner substantial economic savings. This, in turn, can allow countries to invest in greater prevention and health promotion efforts as well as better monitoring and surveillance strategies.

Without question, chronic disease conditions pose the most serious threats to global health. Estimates suggest that continued traditional care of these conditions on a global level will result in cumulative economic losses exceeding $7 trillion between the years of 2011 and 2025.[124] These are staggering figures. This is a strong incentive for changes in policies and strategies that might reduce chronic disease burdens throughout the world, and improving the availability and affordability of technologies can facilitate attaining this goal. As one might expect, the WHO has identified technology as an area of importance as well.[125]

Major Global Health Conditions

In an effort to define optimal strategies for better global health management, as well as potential technologies and solutions, we'll take a closer look at major global health conditions. In doing so, we can better appreciate the magnitude of the problem, as well as identify lifestyle areas and others where interventions may be needed. Some of the most significant conditions affecting global health today are hypertension, obesity, diabetes, and cardiovascular disease.

---

123   Ibid.
124   Ibid.
125   Ibid.

Hypertension has long been recognized as a highly prevalent condition as well as a health disorder linked to a number of other health conditions. Overall, hypertension results in nearly ten million deaths per year, with a total prevalence of 22 percent throughout the world. This makes it one of the most common poor health conditions, and low- to middle-income nations are often hit the hardest. By definition, hypertension is present when either the systolic pressure exceeds 140mm or the diastolic pressure exceeds 90mm. Untreated elevation above these figures has been associated with a number of other illnesses, including heart attack, stroke, vascular dementia, renal impairment, retinal disease, and congestive heart failure. Thus, targeting hypertensive treatment can have beneficial effects downstream.[126]

Interventions can be separated into different tiers. One tier identifies risk factors for hypertension, reflecting an effort in prevention. Specific risk factors include alcohol use, lack of physical activity, obesity, excessive sodium and fat intake, psychological stress, and lack of education. Likewise, limited access to blood pressure monitoring devices and overall care is an additional risk factor. A lack of financial resources, trained personnel, or the devices themselves may contribute to the problem. Access issues are typically much worse in lower socioeconomic nations.[127]

In addition to addressing behavior and access factors, drug therapy and adherence to these treatments represent another major tier for combating hypertension. Generally, drug therapy is indicated for a systolic blood pressure above 160mm and/or a diastolic blood pressure above 100mm. Likewise, drug therapy may be indicated when lower levels of hypertension fail to respond to lifestyle and behavioral measures. Of course, drug therapy is more costly, but when compared to a lack of treatment with subsequent complications, this option is by far more cost effective. For example, the costs of coronary artery

---

126   Ibid.
127   Ibid.

bypass surgery, renal dialysis, and carotid artery surgery are significantly more than drug therapy. In addition, drug therapy is effective. A drop of 10mm in systolic blood pressure with treatment is associated with a 22 percent reduction in coronary artery disease risk and a 41 percent reduction in stroke risk.[128]

Given these benefits with treatment, encouraging proper screening and care of hypertension should be encouraged and incentivized. Unfortunately, a fifth of the world population is unaware they have elevated blood pressure. Even among those who are aware, only half are controlled with treatments, and a quarter of those diagnosed continue to be untreated.[129] In addition to behavior and drug therapy, involving individuals in their own monitoring and care is critical. Self-care and self-monitoring reduces burdens on healthcare system access pressures, and it reflects a more cost-effective, preventive approach to treatment. This is where technologies may play a significant role.

A second major global health issue involves obesity. This epidemic has affected all higher-income nations to some extent. Overall, nearly 3.5 million deaths occur annually due to excess weight. Best estimates suggest 40 percent of all adults worldwide are either overweight or obese, and this percentage has doubled over the past three decades. In addition, over half a billion of the world's population is obese—11 percent of all men and 15 percent of all women.[130]

By definition, obesity is defined as having a body mass index (BMI) 30 kg/m2 or more, while an overweight person by definition has a BMI between 25 and 30 kg/m2. Both of these conditions are associated with advanced risks for several serious health conditions, including diabetes mellitus, hypertension, heart disease, stroke, sleep apnea, osteoarthritis, reduced fertility, and some cancers, such as

---

128   Ibid.
129   Ibid.
130   Ibid.

colon cancer.[131] In addition, the rate of overweight or obese children has also increased dramatically, with over a third of children now falling within this category. More importantly, early childhood obesity is linked to both adult obesity and premature cardiovascular disease.[132] Addressing this health condition has far-reaching ramifications.

This epidemic strikes some countries more than others. For example, countries in the Americas have the highest rates of being overweight and obese, with 61 percent of the population overweight and 27 percent obese. European and Eastern Mediterranean areas approach these figures as well. The lowest rates occur in Southeast Asian nations, with an average obesity rate of 5 percent.[133] Understanding that women and higher income nations are at greater risk for obesity, we can better develop targeted strategies to address this health issue.

Ideal BMI levels of a population should average between 21 and 23 kg/m2, and several potential causes have been identified. Education and policies that create disincentives to eat high calorie foods could prove helpful, while also encouraging fruits, vegetables, and fiber. Another strategy seeks to limit the number of hours a person is sedentary during the course of the day. Combining these efforts with ways to encourage physical activity is important. Strategies to achieve these goals range from various education and awareness campaigns to taxation on some food products.[134] At the same time, many software applications are becoming increasingly popular that encourage activity and healthy diets. This may reflect great opportunities to evoke change and promote health through better use of existing resources.

The prevalence of diabetes mellitus is also relevant to global health concerns. Overall, diabetes accounts for 1.5 million deaths per year, and this condition affects 9 percent of the global population. While

---

131   Ibid.
132   Centers for Disease Control (CDC), "Childhood obesity facts," 2015, https://www.cdc.gov/healthyschools/obesity/facts.htm.
133   WHO, 2014.
134   Ibid.

this condition tends to be most common in countries with higher socioeconomic status, the rates of diabetes in lower to middle income nations have also been rising. In addition, the aging of the existing population makes diabetes more common also since glucose intolerance advances with age. In addition, reduced physical activity and obesity contribute to the rise of diabetes in both higher and lower income regions.[135]

Diabetes mellitus is classically defined as a fasting serum glucose of 126 mg/dl or higher. While the condition is associated with genetic risks and aging, it is also associated with many modifiable risk factors. In fact, the majority of diabetic-related deaths can be prevented through healthy diet and physical activity measures. This is important not only for strategy development but also for reducing other conditions associated with diabetes. Diabetes is known to heighten the risk of coronary artery disease, stroke, renal disease, hypertension, loss of sight, and limb amputation. By targeting modifiable factors like diet, exercise, and effective weight management, the prevalence of these other conditions would decline as well.[136]

A number of strategies have been identified to reduce the prevalence of diabetes. One target area relates to food production. Research shows that subsidies and policies that promote the production of fruits, vegetables, and healthy foods at the expense of unhealthy ones can be effective in reducing diabetic risk. Some countries have even banned specific unhealthy foods completely with positive results. These strategies, along with tax relief programs for healthy food producers, reflect one main area of interest.[137]

A second strategy relates to consumption choices. Nutritional labeling and consumer information are important. Specifically, front-of-package labels that identify key nutritional contents facilitate better

---

135   Ibid.
136   Ibid.
137   Ibid.

consumer choice, as do point-of-purchase information on restaurant menus. Also, pricing strategies, again through tax relief plans and subsidies, can encourage healthy food selections by lowering the price of these foodstuffs compared to unhealthy ones. Finally, several nations have adopted bans and restrictions on advertising, particularly the marketing of unhealthy foods to children, to reduce diabetes as well as obesity.[138]

The other strategy recommended to reduce diabetic risk relates to the environment itself. Work, school, and community organizational settings that favor healthy activity and diet can enhance and support messages of media health campaigns. Already evident in school settings, extending these strategies into other settings outside the home would be welcomed also.[139] By saturating individuals' environments with continued positive messages about healthy lifestyle choices, the prevalence of diabetes would likely decline significantly.

The other major consideration in terms of global health conditions involves cardiovascular disease. Overall, a reported 17.5 million deaths occurred in 2012 from cardiovascular disease, with slightly more of these attributed to heart attacks than strokes. Interestingly, in higher income countries, better drug management and reduction in risks among the populations have resulted in a reduction of cardiovascular disease. However, in lower income countries, the risk is climbing, making it a key disease target for improved global health. Likewise, cardiovascular disease still ranks in the top three conditions of all-cause mortality in the world.[140]

Strategies to reduce cardiovascular disease involve identifying vulnerable regions and individuals and adopting policies to assist these populations. But unlike some of the other conditions discussed, further reduction in cardiovascular disease prevalence has proven to

---

138   Ibid.
139   Ibid.
140   Ibid.

not only be attainable but also affordable. Education and drug therapy can easily be provided to all nations throughout the world. As a result, efforts to reach all individuals, especially in low income areas, should be a priority. Technologies offer a potential medium to facilitate education as well as provider access and guidance.

Many chronic noncommunicable global health diseases can be modified through better individual education, awareness, and incentives. Through these efforts, people worldwide can make healthier lifestyle choices. We will discuss strategies relative to these areas of interest in addition to areas where technology might be advantageous in attaining objectives.

Strategies to Enhance Better Lifestyle Choices

Several strategies targeting specific health factors, and associated public policies, have been suggested to combat chronic noncommunicable disease. Obvious lifestyle choices that lead to chronic disease conditions include tobacco use, alcohol use, lack of physical activity, and a poor diet. Through education, better monitoring, and even structural effects, technologies can provide a means by which health goals become more likely.[141] We'll consider key strategies for several health areas.

One area where such strategies have been considered involves the use of alcohol. Alcohol use has been associated with a number of chronic conditions. While liver cirrhosis and pancreatitis are well recognized, several cancers are also linked to excessive alcohol consumption, including oral, pharyngeal, esophageal, liver, colon, rectal, and breast cancers. In addition, alcohol use is associated with higher risks for cardiovascular disease. In 2012, nearly 6 percent of all deaths were alcohol related, and of these, half were associated with some

---

141   Ibid.

form of chronic disease.[142] Therefore, strategies that reduce alcohol use favor better global health.

Interestingly, alcohol use increases as the overall economic status of a nation increases. Thus, developed nations tend to have higher rates of alcohol consumption compared to developing nations, and they likewise have higher numbers of alcohol-related health disorders. This fact offers some insights into how public policies can influence behaviors related to alcohol use in these nations. For example, policies that make access to alcohol more difficult through taxation and regulatory restrictions deter alcohol use and promote better health. Likewise, policies that limit or ban alcohol beverage advertising can also be effective. At the same time, health services should offer prevention education as well as treatment services.[143] Technology may provide a more efficient and effective way to implement policy change.

Another key strategy to enhance global health involves augmenting physical activity among individuals. Guidelines encourage at least 150 minutes weekly, or twenty minutes daily, of moderate to intense exercise for adults, and sixty minutes daily for children ages five to seventeen years. Achieving these targets is associated with a reduction in risk of a number of chronic conditions, including cardiovascular disease, diabetes mellitus, cancer, and overall mortality. In addition, physical activity promotes health in a number of bodily systems. In addition to lung and cardiovascular structures, muscles, bones, metabolism, and mental health are all enhanced with higher levels of physical activity.[144]

Unfortunately, a sizable portion of the global population fails to meet these targets. Based on surveys from 2010, approximately a fifth of all adult men and over a quarter of all adult women did not meet

---

142   Ibid.
143   Ibid.
144   Ibid.

physical activity guidelines targets. The overall prevalence for inadequate physical activity for adults was 32 percent. For adolescents, the findings were even worse. Among all teens from eleven to seventeen years, more than three-quarters of all boys and five out of every six girls failed to have adequate physical activity. And in terms of overall mortality, poor physical activity accounted for 3.2 million deaths that year.[145] Not only does this suggest a need for health strategies in this area, but interventions could potentially have a significant impact.

In terms of specific recommendations concerning physical activity incentives, certainly education and awareness campaigns can be effective. Various public health advertising programs have proven beneficial in increasing activity levels, particularly among children. However, public policies need to also address a child's environment as a means to encourage greater physical activity. In countries where the setting offers high walkability opportunities, the likelihood that physical activity targets could be met increased by 12 percent. In addition, these increases were unrelated to overall income levels, indicating environmental effects act independently to encourage exercise.[146]

As nations develop, they develop increasing dependence on automobiles, and this can negatively affect levels of physical activity. In addition, automobiles lead to traffic congestion, which means more time spent seated behind the wheel. And such traffic leads to other negative health factors such as carbon emissions, air pollution, noise pollution, and vehicular accidents. Strategies that seek to change the environment along with education and awareness campaigns appear to be the most effective in encouraging physical activity.[147] The use of various technologies (including GPS devices, ride-sharing data systems, bicycle rental inventories, and more) can also help facilitate these efforts.

---

145   Ibid.
146   Ibid.
147   Ibid.

Another area of concern involves the amount of salt and sodium individuals consume. High levels of sodium consumption have been linked to a number of health conditions, including hypertension, cardiovascular disease, and stroke. In assessing the potential impact such a strategy may have, baseline levels demonstrate that sodium intake currently is excessive, on average. While the recommended amount of sodium consumed daily should be around 2 grams, the average level of consumption is closer to 5 grams. In addition, roughly 1.7 million deaths per year have been associated with high sodium intake.[148] Therefore, strategies that reduce sodium consumption have great potential for improving health, and they have also been found to be some of the most cost-effective endeavors.

While all countries may benefit from these strategies regarding sodium, middle- to high-income nations have the highest intake of sodium on average. Therefore, the impact may be greater in these countries. Key areas where efforts should be invested include public awareness campaigns, since voluntary sodium restriction has been shown to respond to educational efforts. In addition, countries should adopt policies that favor effective food labeling so consumers can accurately make determinations about the sodium content of their foods. This should extend into restaurant and catering areas as well through public and private sector collaborations. And food industry organizations and manufacturers should similarly participate in such policies in order to make the strongest impact. Through these efforts, a defined national target sodium consumption amount, and ongoing science and research, nations can effectively align population sodium consumption with desired levels.[149]

Among the most notable lifestyle choice involving health is the decision to abstain from tobacco use and, if possible, to avoid secondhand smoke. Overall, more than six million deaths per year are attributed to

---

148   Ibid.
149   Ibid.

tobacco use, and this includes over 600,000 from secondhand smoke and 170,000 children. Tobacco use has been linked to a variety of poor health conditions, including cardiovascular disease, respiratory illnesses, several cancers, stroke, and diabetes. Yet despite this fact and public awareness campaigns, 7 percent of all deaths in men and 12 percent of women can be attributed to tobacco use. And 37 percent of all men and 7 percent of all women smoke tobacco, with the vast majority smoking daily. This equates to 1.1 billion people globally, identifying tobacco use as a major area of health concern.[150]

In addition to awareness campaigns and ongoing patient education, many additional efforts can be taken to further reduce tobacco use. Proven strategies in some countries have involved expanding the size of the health labels and warnings on packages. Some almost encompass the entire packaging material. Some countries even ban the use of a logo on packages, with additional restrictions on the use of various symbols and caricatures. Likewise, bans or severe restrictions on advertising and sponsorship abilities of tobacco projects is also a commonly promoted health strategy which has had positive effects concurrently with antitobacco ad campaigns. Last, as with other lifestyle incentives strategies, increased taxes on tobacco products deter tobacco use, with many countries having tax rates as high as 80 percent. Such approaches have demonstrated effectiveness and should be considered in further reducing the prevalence of tobacco use.

Global health requires continued efforts to reach a variety of populations in deterring poor lifestyles choices and enhancing positive ones. Those choices that have the most significant impact on global health deserve the most attention as well as the investment of the majority of resources available. Likewise, ongoing surveillance and research to determine the effects of these strategies can help better refine future efforts to enhance global health. And while many traditional strategies

---

150   Ibid.

are effective, new technologies offer the opportunity to enhance these efforts even further.

Summary Thoughts

In examining the overall picture concerning global health, major challenges lie ahead: aging populations, limited access to healthcare services, factors negatively influencing lifestyle choices, and limited financial resources. Targeting conditions that affect the most number of people and have the highest associated death and morbidity rates are important in developing effective strategies. Likewise, we should seek strategies proven to be effective, affordable, and efficient.

Access to drugs and technologies are of significant importance in effectively monitoring, evaluating, and managing global health moving forward. This means facilitating the production, procurement, and distribution of generic medications that can be used to treat target diseases by all populations. A number of essential medication classes used to treat hypertension, diabetes, lipid disorders, respiratory illnesses, and cardiovascular disease should be considered in this regard.[151] Policies should be pursued to advance access to these medications for all countries and regions.

At the same time, we should pursue technologies to help manage these conditions globally. Basic technologies that should be available for all individuals include devices that can measure blood pressure, height, weight, blood glucose, cholesterol levels, and albumin levels in the urine.[152] These technologies allow greater self-monitoring and care, which can alleviate pressures on access demands. Exploring the use of telemedicine and other informatics technologies within healthcare could offer additional solutions to healthcare access

---

151 Ibid.
152 Ibid.

issues.[153] Through evidenced-based practice guidelines, and through patient-centered care, these information technologies should be evaluated for their efficacy in helping solve these global health issues.

---

153   Ibid.

CHAPTER 5

Health Information Technologies

Healthcare has come a long way over the last few decades in using technology. In contrast to the use of traditional patient records such as paper charts, handwritten prescriptions, and standardized paper order forms, today's healthcare system has adopted many digital paperless platforms to aid in storage demands, efficiency, and standardizations as well as documentation. But healthcare still lags behind other industry sectors, and it also faces unique challenges when it comes to using healthcare information technologies (HITs) in the most optimal way. In this chapter, we will discuss the current state of HIT and its potential challenges in addition to future anticipated directions.

The concept of HIT encompasses a wide array of devices, software packages, and systems that utilize digital technologies to store, display, file, catalog, analyze, communicate, and utilize healthcare information. For example, HIT includes not only electronic health records (EHR) but also personal health records (PHR), computerized physician order entry (CPOE), physician support systems (PSS), picture archiving and communication systems (PACS), and data management systems. It also includes the use of the Internet, social media, desktop computers, laptops, smartphones, tablets, and a host of other potential communications and devices.

Examining all aspects of HIT is certainly beyond the scope of this chapter as well as this book. However, we'll explore the current state of EHR usage, and HIT pitfalls and challenges. Likewise, it is also important to explore future expectations related to HIT, including the advancing role telemedicine and telehealth may play moving forward. Through examining these specific HIT areas, we will gain a better understanding of potential solutions for national and global healthcare issues.

HITECH and Meaningful Use

The Health Information Technology for Economic and Clinical Health (HITECH) Act was established as part of Title VII of the American Recovery and Reinvestment Act of 2009. HITECH not only incentivized providers to implement EHR as part of their patient care system, but likewise it served to penalize providers receiving Medicare if implementation and meaningful use was not eventually adopted.[154] Likewise, many private health insurers followed this lead and developed a pay for performance plan for EHR meaningful use as well.[155]

The goal of HITECH was to improve care coordination among providers, engage patients and families in health issues and care, improve public health, and ensure continued privacy and security of health information. Phased implementation of HITECH requirements involved different stages of meaningful use that providers had to adopt. Core requirements during the initial phase involved CPOE, e-prescribing, medication and allergy interaction checks, health information chart updates, Clinical Decision Support Systems (CDSS) tools, quality measure reporting, and others. These requirements placed significant pressures on providers to adopt EHR in specific ways in order to maintain financial viability.[156]

---

154   Ashish K. Jha, "Health information technology comes of age: comment on 'Achieving meaningful use of health information technology,'" *Archives of Internal Medicine* 172, no. 9 (2012): 737–738.
155   Pam Arlotto, "7 strategies for improving HITECH readiness: demonstrating meaningful use of electronic health records is critical in an environment of outcome-based payment and healthcare reform. CFOs will be vital to this initiative," *Healthcare Financial Management* 64, no. 11 (2010): 90–96.
156   Jha, 2012.

HITECH has been beneficial in many regards, including easier access to patient information, enhanced measures of safety regarding medication checks, electronic reminders to aid clinical data collection, and greater efficiency in transferring of patient information. Negatives, however, have involved the cost of the EHR system itself, training costs related to time investments, temporary reduplication of resource investments, and frustrations during implementation phases.[157] To some extent, financial incentives within HITECH for providers eased the financial pressures. Additionally, better information regarding patients and enhanced collaboration among providers hoped to improve efficiency of care, reduce care delays, avoid late developing complications, and reduce reduplication costs.[158]

While Phase I of HITECH was based on meaningful use of EHR among providers from a predominantly clinical perspective, subsequent phases addressed the meaningful use of EHR to develop enhanced quality of healthcare from both clinical and economic perspectives. Therefore providers were encouraged to develop a vision that supported new healthcare models utilizing EHR. Likewise, expanding models of health information exchange between providers and patients were required. Meaningful use of EHR has thus evolved, and is still evolving.[159]

The Electronic Health Records Experience

A little more than a decade ago, roughly 10 percent of physicians used EHR systems. This figure has dramatically changed, however. Today approximately 70 percent of providers now have adopted EHR use with nearly eight in ten physicians in office practices making the transition from paper to digital records. In addition, roughly a third

---

157   Ibid.
158   Arlotto, 2010.
159   Ibid.

of all doctors have fully functional EHR systems that incorporate patient charts with imaging, testing, and physician ordering components.[160] With the passage of HITECH and incentives based through meaningful use policies, a fairly rapid shift toward EHR adoption has occurred.

In terms of meaningful use, three-quarters of physicians who use EHR meet meaningful use criteria. Between 2011 and 2014, this generated nearly $23 billion incentive payments for physicians under HITECH guidelines. However, EHR adoption is not without significant costs. By far, EHR investments are the largest HIT investments physicians make, and an estimated $37 billion was spent in EHR costs alone during 2014. In addition, high levels of dissatisfaction exist among physicians and healthcare administrators with the EHR systems they currently have. Forty percent of administrators and two-thirds of physicians gave EHR low ratings.[161]

In considering the potential positive advantages of EHR adoption, areas of efficiency, safety, and quality have been touted. First, EHR allows more efficient data collection and storage, which in turn permits information to be more readily transferred or transmitted among different providers. EHR allows patient records to be remotely accessed as well, which can enhance patient care, avoid duplication of services, and speed up services. In addition, incentives related to chart documentation within EHR exist, since this allows better compliance with medical standards while reducing legal malpractice risks. Likewise, better documentation helps support medical billing practices while maximizing reimbursement for actual services rendered.[162] Each of these is valuable from a physician's perspective.

Other potential benefits with EHR involve the ability to reduce medical errors. Overall, medical errors account for nearly $20

---

160   Ryan Shay, "EHR adoption rates: 19 must-see stats," *Practice Fusion Blog*, 2016, http://www.practicefusion.com/blog/ehr-adoption-rates/.
161   Ibid.
162   Nir Menachemi and Taleah H. Collum, "Benefits and drawbacks of electronic health record systems," *Risk Management and Healthcare Policy* 4 (2011): 47–55.

billion a year in medical costs and represent the third leading cause of death.[163] EHR has the capacity to significantly reduce such errors through better documentation, better legibility, enhanced information access, and internal safety checks. For example, e-prescribing abilities associated with an EHR system can compare prescription data to medications a patient takes, patient allergies, drug interactions, and duplicate prescriptions while also guiding physicians on what safety information should be relayed to the patient. And similarly, CDSSs offer improvements in patient safety and care by enabling point-of-care access to evidence-based practice guidelines and research.[164] Through these benefits, quality as well as costs are improved.

The aforementioned advantages of EHR certainly sound attractive to a healthcare system with excessive expenditures and inefficiencies. However, the use of EHR in actual practice has not yet realized these advantages to the fullest extent. For individual physicians, the costs of investing in HIT systems are substantial, and being able to account for these investments through future earnings is a challenge. While the incentives under meaningful use help, cost remains a significant obstacle since ongoing investments are needed over time as technologies advance. Despite the potential advantages EHR offers, financial realities can undermine the benefits.

A second issue that has affected full adoption and satisfaction with EHR among physicians relates to use of EHR in comparison to traditional patient care measures. In essence, physicians were placed in a position of data entry once EHR systems became the norm. Rather than taking abbreviated notes and dictating medical records for transcription, physicians now enter data directly into electronic patient charts and files. Despite the use of assistants and nursing staff to facilitate this process, evidence supports that this task significantly impacts physician time. In some cases, patient care and workflow

---

163   Shay, 2016.
164   Menachemi, 2011.

times have been doubled for doctors using EHR. While point-of-care and bedside systems are less impactful when compared to centralized or office-based computers, significant delays remain.[165] This is a major reason for dissatisfaction with many EHR systems.

One of the major proposed benefits of EHR is reduction in the duplication of healthcare services through more effective information sharing. However, in reality, these redundancies have been replaced by others. Many physicians in using EHR systems often will enter duplicate information from other sources into the EHR record. Many systems likewise offer copy and paste options, and physicians often perform this function in an effort to save time. Thus effective documentation to support medical decisions and billing practices is often excessive, redundant, and unnecessary. The end result of these practices is patient documents and charts that are not only saturated with repeated information, but also inefficiencies in chart reviews and data access. Because physicians and other providers must filter through the "data noise," any potential time savings using EHR are lost.

The last issue that has undermined EHR success to date involves the inability of information sharing among different systems. Over 1,100 EHR vendors currently exist, and this figure has doubled in the last four years.[166] In the next section, this subject of poor interoperability will be discussed in greater detail. Based on these issues, HITs do not always provide a magic solution for all the ailments of a fragmented, highly regulated, inefficient healthcare system. However, EHR and HITs do offer the potential to solve many of the existing problems if utilized in effective ways. The challenge involves defining and verifying these methods of use so healthcare to optimize resources as well as outcomes.

---

165   Lise Poissant, Jennifer Pereira, Robyn Tamblyn, and Yuko Kawasumi, "The impact of electronic health records on time efficiency of physicians and nurses: a systematic review," *Journal of the American Medical Informatics Association* 12, no. 5 (2005): 505–516.
166   Shay, 2016.

Interoperability and HIT Challenges

Regarding HIT, one of the most notable issues involves interoperability. Interoperability can be defined as the ability to exchange, understand, and act on patient and other health-related information among diverse systems and organizations in an effort to enhance collaboration and efficiency.[167] Unfortunately, success in pursuing interoperability in healthcare has proven to be challenging for a number of reasons despite the potential benefits it might offer.

In the US, healthcare expenditures now exceed 17 percent of the nation's gross domestic product, and billions of dollars are spent on a system that is notably fragmented and inefficient. Interoperability has been identified as a potential solution to reduce such costs. Estimates in this regard suggest that $77 billion could be saved annually from this advancement alone. It therefore stands to reason that benefits and challenges to interoperability deserve attention as the nation strives to address healthcare services to an aging population and a rising chronic disease burden.[168]

Over the course of the last few decades, the US healthcare system has developed in a diverse and fragmented manner. Independent vendors and providers have contributed to this fragmentation by developing and utilizing various health informatics systems, respectively, in a disjointed manner. For example, vendors developed EHR systems, health administrative systems, and other software unilaterally without any degree of collaboration with other vendors. Likewise, hospitals and physicians have purchased and used an array of informatics systems. In fact, dozens of different systems may be utilized within one organization without any capacity for the systems to communicate

---

167   Patrick Kierkegaard, "Interoperability after deployment: persistent challenges and regional strategies in Denmark," *International Journal for Quality in Health Care* 27, no. 2 (2015).

168   Olaronke Iroju, Abimbola Soriyan, Ishaya Gambo, and Janet Olaleke, "Interoperability in healthcare: benefits, challenges and resolutions," *International Journal of Innovation and Applied Studies* 3, no. 1 (2013): 262–270.

with one another. As a result, information sharing is inhibited, and health decisions are made without a full complement of knowledge regarding individual patients.[169]

Understanding this environment, the potential impact that greater interoperability may provide is intuitive. When systems are better able to share information regarding patients throughout and between organizations, those organizations can provide more comprehensive care. From the standpoint of quality, healthcare decisions can be made based on a full complement of data rather than on limited information. From a cost perspective, enhanced patient safety and reduced duplication of testing and evaluations can result when better information sharing exists. And from an accessibility standpoint, interoperability facilitates better patient data access to all providers, which promotes greater collaboration. These areas can make a tremendous impact not only on individual patient care but on the entire healthcare system as a whole.[170]

Other potential benefits related to better interoperability involve the ability to use big data and data analytics. With integration of healthcare information regarding an array of patients and systems, knowledge regarding optimal care practices can be gained as a result. This has notable implications on chronic disease care in addition to care related to specific populations. With such abilities, better clinical guidelines and policies can be developed, again enhancing efficiency and quality of care. And at the same time, resource utilization can be improved, along with lower expenditures.[171] Given these potential advantages, the pursuit of interoperability seems logical.

The most obvious challenge in pursuing interoperability stems from gaining vendor support. In order to achieve interoperability, vendors

---

169   Shalini Bhartiya and Deepti Mehrotra, "Exploring interoperability approaches and challenges in healthcare data exchange," *International Conference on Smart Health*, (Springer Berlin Heidelberg, 2013) 52–65.

170   Iroju, 2013.

171   Jens Weber-Jahnke, Liam Peyton, and Thodoros Topaloglou, "eHealth system interoperability," *Information Systems Frontiers* 14, no. 1 (2012): 1–3.

may feel at risk for giving away trade secrets or competitive advantages. In addition, legacy systems in place may not even be able to achieve interoperability with more recent HIT systems. Other challenges relate simply to the complexity of healthcare itself. Healthcare coding has numerous inconsistencies between terminologies and clinical states, and developing standards as well as accurate informational terms poses practical problems.[172] These issues stand in the way of allowing interoperability to aid healthcare functions overall.

Though these challenges exist, the development of health information exchanges that permit interoperability and information sharing remain an obvious focus. The Office of the National Coordinator for Health Information Technologies is pursuing national standards to ensure compliance with a single system. In order to achieve meaningful use of EHR and HIT, interoperability is an essential ingredient. Therefore, continued progress will likely be made in this direction in the immediate future.

Telemedicine and the Future of HIT

Our focus on HIT systems thus far has been on reducing healthcare costs, enhancing quality of care, and enhancing efficiency and patient outcomes through electronic health records (EHRs). However, several other HITs are being utilized in an attempt to achieve major healthcare objectives as well. Of these, telemedicine represents one HIT that has tremendous potential in healthcare and may ultimately serve as a disruptive innovation that changes the entire system.

Telemedicine, as understood today, dates back to the late 1960s. In 1968, the use of telemedicine was used in Massachusetts to link a medical care clinic at Boston's Logan Airport to Massachusetts General Hospital.[173] Since that time, telemedicine has gradually become

---

172   Bhartiya, 2013.
173   Rashid L. Bashshur, Gary W. Shannon, Brian R. Smith, Dale C. Alverson, Nina Antoniotti, William G. Barsan, Noura Bashshur, et al., "The empirical foundations of telemedicine interventions for chronic disease management," *Telemedicine and e-Health* 20, no. 9 (2014): 769–800.

more commonplace, and today, more than half of all hospital systems currently have some type of telemedicine or telehealth program. Advances in telecommunications, broadband Internet, and mobile devices have all facilitated these changes. Likewise, telemedicine is used in a variety of health conditions ranging from women's health to specialty pediatric care, neurological care, cardiac evaluations, mental health, urgent care services, and many others. In particular, telemedicine has been identified as a potential means to service rural areas without a broad scope of services to enhance and reduce the cost of quality care.[174]

Unfortunately, many terms are often used interchangeably to describe telemedicine. Common ones include telehealth, e-health, health telematics, telecare, and others. For the purpose of this discussion, telemedicine refers to the provision of healthcare services, clinical information, and health education over a geographic distance utilizing telecommunication technologies in order to provide some means of patient care. In contrast, telehealth, though often used synonymously with telemedicine, will refer to the same actions in a more general sense in order to promote or protect the health of individuals and communities at large. Last, e-health refers to the delivery of electronic health information, education, commercial products, and/or commercial services over the Internet by healthcare professionals and nonprofessionals alike.[175] Each of these areas is relevant to the use of technologies in healthcare, and each reflects different opportunities and platforms as well.

While many hospitals and healthcare systems have adopted the use of telemedicine over the past couple of decades, the history concerning the regulatory environment surrounding telemedicine reflects a typical

---

174   Jeremy M. Kahn, "Virtual visits—confronting the challenges of telemedicine," *New England Journal of Medicine* 372, no. 18 (2015): 1684–1685.

175   Farhad Fatehi and Richard Wootton, "Telemedicine, telehealth or e-health? A bibliometric analysis of the trends in the use of these terms," *Journal of Telemedicine and Telecare* 18, no. 8 (2012): 460–464.

lag. For example, the Center for Medicare Services (CMS) failed to recognize telemedicine until 1997 when the Balanced Budget Act was passed, and even then, the use of telemedicine was constrained until later changes in 2001. Even after this, telemedicine has been recognized only in its applications related to video consultation without consideration of other potential health services applications. Because of this, Medicare has lagged behind the technological potential of telemedicine as well as its potential regarding enhanced healthcare services.[176]

Despite limitations described at regulatory levels, private and public health organizations and systems have adopted certain telemedicine technologies. Today, many hospitals, both urban and rural, have telemedicine programs and service a wide variety of populations. While the primary use still involves video consultation, many other uses are either in place or are being considered. Examples of these other uses include remote outpatient monitoring, patient health education services, continuing medical education for professionals, and rehabilitation support programs.[177] Likewise, telemedicine is being used by many different health disciplines, including neurology, oncology, obstetrics, emergency care, cardiology, pulmonology, pediatrics, and critical care in both outpatient and inpatient settings. And organizations such as home healthcare, nursing homes, and other visiting health services are increasingly employing telemedicine in specific contexts.[178]

Several aspects of today's healthcare system are encouraging for the use of telemedicine today. Telemedicine has the potential to reduce healthcare costs by reducing patient and provider travel, decreasing

176   M. G. Gaynor, "Evaluation of patient to provider oriented telemedicine in hospitals and physician practices," *Muskie School of Public Service Capstone Paper 103, University Southern Maine*, (2015), 1–31.
177   Curtis L. Lowery, Janet M. Bronstein, Tina L. Benton, and David A. Fletcher, "Distributing medical expertise: the evolution and impact of telemedicine in Arkansas," *Health Affairs* 33, no. 2 (2014): 235–243.
178   David C. Grabowski and A. James O'Malley, "Use of telemedicine can reduce hospitalizations of nursing home residents and generate savings for Medicare," *Health Affairs* 33, no. 2 (2014): 244–250.

physical resources (such as office space), and shifting care away from high-cost centers (such as hospitals and emergency rooms). At the same time, telemedicine has the potential to offer enhanced quality of care through greater access. This is generally most beneficial for rural communities without access to specialized care, incarcerated individuals, and elderly with limited mobility options.[179]

In most instances, however, patients must still access a location that has been equipped and, in most cases, certified as a telemedicine center. Center approval for telemedicine use relates to reimbursement requirements by third-party payers; therefore, home-based telemedicine is not necessarily common.[180] As a result, individuals may still have to travel to a physician's office, outpatient clinic, or other facility to gain access to the benefits telemedicine offers. More aggressive states have encouraged the development of telemedicine sites while others have not.[181] This reflects an area where change is evolving as information and evidence become more available.

Like EHR systems, a major challenge to implementing telemedicine involves costs. Implementing telemedicine thus can vary depending on the size of the organization, the outreach of services, the quality of the system, and other variables. Similarly, reimbursement issues are also noteworthy since nearly all third-party payers, including Medicare and Medicaid, only recognize video consultation as a reimbursable service with telemedicine. Patient monitoring and other telemedicine uses may not be covered.[182] Because of these financial issues, rapid adoption of telemedicine has lagged behind some other HIT opportunities.

Last, interstate regulations and requirements have also deterred rapid adoption of telemedicine. Telemedicine naturally allows the

179   Kahn, 2015.
180   Tim B. Hunter, Ronald S. Weinstein, and Elizabeth A. Krupinski, "State medical licensure for telemedicine and teleradiology," *Telemedicine and e-Health* 21, no. 4 (2015): 315–318.
181   Lowery, 2014.
182   Ibid.

extension of healthcare services across state lines as well as across national boundaries. However, current state laws regarding telemedicine require a provider to be licensed in the state where the patient receives care. In other words, if telemedicine services involve twenty-five different states, then a physician would be required to have a license in all of them. Not only does this result in significant financial costs to the physician, but the time required to acquire all of these licenses is tremendous.[183]

The potential that telemedicine has in the areas mentioned is certainly substantial, but policy change and regulatory change at federal and state levels will be required for this potential to be better realized. This is particularly important for global health issues in addition to national ones. Imagine low- to middle-income countries having access to specialists throughout the world through remote telemedicine technologies. Access to care would be tremendously better, and the cost savings resulting from the avoidance of infrastructure and resource development would be significant. Naturally, such technology would augment patient quality of care as well as safety on a global scale. But many financial and political barriers will need to change. If barriers can be broken, which inevitably should be based on resource availability alone, then telemedicine may well be one of the greatest disruptive innovations within HIT.

Telemedicine not only may improve access and quality care but may also facilitate self-management and self-care as well. Remote sharing of data and information could allow better monitoring of chronic conditions like diabetes, hypertension, and chronic respiratory dysfunction. Likewise, patients could receive state-of-the-art education and updates about their conditions, enhancing their own knowledge and ability to oversee aspects of their care. Shifting some self-care monitoring and oversight would be advantageous from a

---

183   Ibid.

resource perspective, and this likewise would enhance patient autonomy and involvement. Thus, telemedicine offers many opportunities to advance overall healthcare systems.

Telemedicine is not the only HIT solution to advance self-monitoring and self-care. Personal health records (PHR) are additional HIT options that engage patients in their own health and healthcare. Specifically, PHRs are repositories of health information maintained by consumers or individuals. In other words, PHRs are similar to EHR systems, but instead of being utilized by physicians and healthcare providers only, PHRs allow patients to enter their own health information and determine which information may be include, shared, and accessed. PHRs also facilitate the ability for patients to be involved in the coordination of their care since they can provide information to various providers about past diagnoses, services, and interventions.[184]

In some instances, PHRs could be used in conjunction with EHR systems. While the integrity of the data and information would be important for review, the potential to reduce data entry time for physicians and to improve information sharing within the healthcare system does exist. By using PHRs in this way, patients become involved in their care to a much greater extent and more knowledgeable at the same time. By definition, PHRs would therefore promote patient-centered care since the patient would have much greater awareness, and at the same time, patients would also be more accountable for their health as a result. This has potential impacts regarding patient choices about lifestyle, diet, and physical activity as well as behaviors regarding adherence to treatments and medical recommendations.[185]

Healthcare systems need to move in the direction of prevention and health promotion instead of being reactionary to disease occurrence. PHRs help encourage such behaviors through active participation of

---

184   Anne Moen and Lina Merete Maeland Knudsen, "Nursing informatics: decades of contribution to health informatics," *Healthcare Informatics Research* 19, no. 2 (2013): 86–92.
185   Ibid.

patients. In addition, greater transparency should similarly develop in the process, enabling patients to better determine the care they want in collaboration with their physicians. Both of these aspects could result in significant healthcare cost savings if greater discernment results along the way. These benefits are particularly important given the expected rise in chronic health illnesses over the next few decades.

A final area of HIT that may affect the future of healthcare involves the expanded use of mobile devices within healthcare systems. In many hospitals and healthcare organizations, the use of mobile devices is met with resistance. The inherent risks associated with security threats to patient health information can affect the willingness to use mobile devices in such settings. Likewise, the costs involved in developing systems that are secure and can accommodate a variety of mobile devices can be daunting. However, the use of such mobile devices in this setting is inevitable. The accessibility, availability, and portability these devices offer is significant, and as these technologies advance, increasing demand to use them within healthcare will occur.[186]

In some parts of the country, surveys have indicated that 98 percent of physicians routinely use their mobile devices in their professional work. At the same time, 75 percent of hospitals are reluctant to allow physicians to connect via these devices to their informatics systems. The risk for privacy information breaches is substantial. In some cases, patients have been rewarded $1,000 each in court because of breaches in security. Likewise, security breaches involving mobile devices often comprise a substantial portion of these instances. With such devices, open viewing of screens pose threats that may be significant in healthcare settings.[187]

---

186   Hays Green, "Strategies for safeguarding security of mobile computing: hospitals can gain a competitive edge by responding strategically to the rapid proliferation of mobile devices in healthcare, with security being an intrinsic part of their strategy," *Healthcare Financial Management* 67, no. 2 (2013): 88–93.
187   Ibid.

Overall, a lack of standardization exists when it comes to implementing "bring your own device" policies and procedures within healthcare. However, several strategies can be pursued as a means to develop such policies while protecting patient privacy and data security. First, organizations should conduct a thorough mobile security risk assessment. This is often performed by third parties and includes firewall analyses, among other assessments. Second, a detailed policy and procedure outline addressing mobile access, storage, transmissions, audits, loss or theft of devices, and responses to breaches represents a best practice. Also, a training program to educate staff about policies and privacy laws is often included as well. And specific measures to reduce unauthorized access using encryption, infrastructure supports, and identity management techniques are typical.[188]

Patient involvement in health management and information systems is already evident, and through the use of cloud computing, social media, mobile applications, and analytics, such involvement is expected to continue to grow. E-health platforms are already in use, as are personal health records. Likewise, over 1.7 billion people downloaded health-related apps for mobile devices, accounting for $26 billion in revenues last year.[189] Through greater access to personal health information and through greater involvement in their healthcare, patients will continue to engage in the coming decades. Healthcare needs to be prepared for these changes and make adjustments and provisions accordingly.

In looking toward the future, the ability for each of the HIT areas to become functional within healthcare systems offers additional hopes. By expanding the use of electronic devices and platforms for health information, the opportunities to use "big data" in healthcare become realistic. With better interoperability, alignment of data from thousands

---

188   Ibid.
189   A. Desai, "Scanning the HIM Environment: AHIMA's 2015 Report Offers Insight on Emerging Industry Trends and Challenges," *Journal of AHIMA*, 86, no. 5 (2015): 38–43.

of healthcare data centers can be combined, stored, and analyzed in order to discover optimal healthcare policies and practices. Such endeavors can identify when and where healthcare resources should be utilized and reveal the benefits patients and systems will receive as a result. Likewise, big data offers promises toward more efficient operations in billing, administration, clinical care, and a number of other areas in healthcare. And such data analysis offers potential rewards in new care and treatment discoveries based on pooled data insights from mass populations as well as advances in computerized decision support systems.[190] As a result, data opportunities may be able to reduce costs, enhance efficiency, and improve quality of care.

Big data management and analytics will be necessary to assist with cost savings in healthcare, better resource utilization, and an assessment of cost-benefit assessments of various interventions. Estimates suggest that big data systems could result in $450 billion in savings alone. Of course, health information exchanges will need to evolve to achieve interoperability in order to accomplish these results, and overcoming interoperability barriers will not be easy.[191] Developing policies, as well as regulatory change that facilitates these policies, will be important, and likewise, must provide the means to fund better interoperability. Despite the challenges, market pressures and ongoing public use of advanced technologies will drive these changes. Therefore, healthcare systems must be ready to adapt accordingly.

With these trends, data security issues and protections will become an increasing concern. In fact, it is estimated that by 2020 almost half of all digital health data will be unprotected. On one hand, this may be inevitable due to the fact that information sharing between systems, providers, and patients is needed. But at the same time, such data needs to be secure, confidential, and private. In addition,

---

190   Joachim Roski, George W. Bo-Linn, and Timothy A. Andrews, "Creating value in health care through big data: opportunities and policy implications," *Health Affairs* 33, no. 7 (2014): 1115–1122.
191   Desai, 2015.

breaches in information security and HIPAA violations have serious implications for physicians and organizations alike.[192] Not only can these be associated with regulatory fines and sanctions, but they can also be associated with disruptions in workflows and negative patient relations. It therefore becomes essential for physicians and healthcare organizations to invest in data security areas as well as other HIT systems in advance.

Summary Considerations

Without question, technology is a driving force in most industries, and over the next several decades, it will continue to drive healthcare as well. In examining recent trends in other sectors, the use of Internet platforms, mobile devices, data analytics, and other tools is certainly becoming more common. These same trends are likely to be seen within healthcare as well, increasing patients' involvement in their care, increasing use of big data, developing mobile health applications and solutions, and advancing health information exchanges and interoperability. These will complement existing structures related to EHR, PHR, and telemedicine, which will similarly advance as well.

HIT systems are the future. In time, these will continue to improve, be more efficient, and incorporate newer features and technologies. HIT systems, however, also have the risk of becoming complicated, expensive, and ultimately to slow down work efficiency while also permitting new sources of medical errors. Communication, collaboration, standardization, and evidence-based research are essential in determining how best to develop these systems and ensure they are truly functional in meeting healthcare needs. These measures along with considerations regarding costs, user training, system support, and systems integration will be required to meet clinical practice needs.

---

192   Desai, 2015.

With these measures considered, higher percentages of adoption and use will occur.

Ultimately, patients should be the recipients of any potential benefits HIT systems provide, and because of this, designs in systems, policies, and use must be patient centered in nature. HIT systems certainly have great potential in enhancing clinical care through ensuring that those who make clinical decisions have proper information and the right tools to render optimal care. At the same time, HIT systems offer advances in efficiency, which can also equate into lower costs and better care outcomes. Naturally, change is difficult, and adopting new HIT systems and workflows pose challenges in any sector. For healthcare, these can be even more significant when resource restraints and data security issues come into play. But with proper development and application, HIT systems offer physicians and patients many advantages and can help remedy many of the current health issues facing the world. And if done successfully, HIT systems can place the emphasis back where it properly belongs . . . on the patient and physician relationship.

CHAPTER 6

ikioo Remote Health Monitoring and Management

The fragmentation and inefficiencies of the US healthcare system have been well documented. Due to a variety of factors, including historical changes, regulatory policies, and reactions to market climates, the system has evolved in a piecemeal, disjointed kind of way. As a result, many aspects of the healthcare system fail to meet target needs while also driving up costs and expenditures. Unnecessary tests, duplicate services, failed follow-up evaluations, and inefficiencies of service continually result in lower quality of care and rising costs. Combine these factors with an aging population with a higher chronic disease burden, and the recipe for tremendous concern is evident.

Everyone experiences delays within the healthcare system. Waiting rooms and areas are labeled such for a reason . . . people spend significant amounts of time waiting. Recent data indicates that the average time spent during a routine medical visit to a physician's office exceeds two hours, and the amount of time lost per visit for an individual equates to about $43 each time.[193] To some extent, some delays are unavoidable since emergencies, urgencies, and the unexpected finding occur without any capacity to predict when or where they might happen. But in other instances, such delays are avoidable. Eliminating these delays can have positive impacts not only in the overall healthcare experience but in the productivity of the nation as

---

193   Jamie Ducharme, "Harvard research says the average medical visit takes 121 minutes," *Boston Magazine*, 2015, http://www.bostonmagazine.com/health/blog/2015/10/12/doctors-appointment-length/.

a whole. Solutions are needed to help reduce, if not eliminate, these unwanted effects.

Another major source of concern related to these healthcare system problems involves the ability to provide effective continuity of care to individuals throughout their life. Let's take a common scenario to demonstrate how such continuity is often lacking. Suppose a patient with diabetes suffers a stroke. The patient is admitted to the hospital where various tests, treatments, and therapies are provided, perhaps without a full knowledge of the patient's prior medical history. The patient is then discharged to a rehabilitative center, which receives only part of the hospital care records, for post-acute care. In addition, a few tests still pending at discharge from the hospital are not reviewed. The patient then goes home with a discharge plan in place. But monitoring of the patient's adherence to the plan is not performed, evaluations of self-care not assessed, and other factors such as psychosocial variables underappreciated. The patient then re-presents to the hospital for readmission three weeks later with poorly controlled diabetes.

Of course, this scenario does not happen all the time, but it occurs more than we realize. In fact, roughly one in five Medicare patients were readmitted to the hospital within a thirty-day period after their original release from the hospital. And unplanned readmissions represent about 17 percent of all hospital costs.[194] These impressive figures highlight the need for better continuity of care and better monitoring of the entire care process. Research has examined hospital readmissions, and on average, more than a quarter have been found to be preventable through better care monitoring and management. The potential impacts regarding healthcare costs and patient quality of care could be significant.

The Affordable Care Act (ACA) introduced the Hospital Readmission Reduction Program (HRRP) in an effort to reduce Medicare

---

194   Eric Alper, Terrence O'Malley, and Jeffery Greenwald, "Hospital discharge and readmission," *UpToDate*, 2016, http://www.uptodate.com/contents/hospital-discharge-and-readmission.

readmissions. Under this program, hospitals were required to meet specific standards regarding readmission rates for specific health conditions. During 2013, the HRRP examined readmission rates within thirty days for patients with heart attack, congestive heart failure, and pneumonia. In 2015, similar rates were examined for chronic obstructive pulmonary disease, total hip replacements, and total knee replacements. Among the 3,400 hospitals participating in the HRRP, less than eight hundred had readmission rates low enough to avoid Medicare reimbursement penalties. The remaining hospitals were subjected to payment reductions ranging from 1 percent to 3 percent depending on how poorly they performed. Based on this recent data, continuity of care and care monitoring are a significant concern.[195]

Failure to properly follow up on pending diagnostic tests represent another area of concern. Based on recent research, approximately 41 percent of patients who were discharged from a hospital had at least one pending test at the time. Likewise, 7 percent of these tests were ordered on the day of discharge. Overall, two-thirds of discharging physicians were unaware such a test was pending, and of the tests ordered on the last admission day, nearly half were never reviewed by the physician.[196]

Understandably, failure to follow up on pending diagnostics at the time of discharge can have negative effects on patient well-being and lead to higher readmission rates as well as other complications. However, the first step in alleviating this problem involves making sure the physician is aware of these pending examinations. In reviewing physicians' discharge summaries, only a quarter tend to mention pending tests, and of the ones that do, a small minority offer a complete list. In addition, tests recommended after discharge are also often not performed. In fact, roughly a third of all post-discharge tests ordered

195   Virgil Dickson, "Hospitals under pressure to cut readmission for minorities, poor," *Modern Healthcare*, 2016, http://www.modernhealthcare.com/article/20160126/NEWS/160129894.
196   Alper, 2016.

or recommended are never completed.[197] Due to failed continuity and a poor mechanism by which adherence monitoring can be performed, a physician's best intentions may fall short.

Patient follow-up after discharge reflects another important area to improve care continuity and quality in healthcare. Often, determining when follow-up should occur requires an assessment of many different variables, including the severity of the patient's illness, the patient's ability to render self-care, physical logistics regarding the care needed, as well as various psychosocial issues. Physician communications, engagement of community care providers, and patient education are well-known areas where patient reevaluations and oversight can be improved. This is another area where remote health management abilities can facilitate better care.

Hospital visits are naturally complex by nature of the heightened disease severity often present. Therefore, the aforementioned statistics may not be surprising. But these figures do indicate key areas where healthcare must improve in order to reduce expenditures and to enhance overall patient outcomes. By 2030, an estimated nearly half of the population will have some type of chronic disease, and the care of these conditions will account for 86 percent of all healthcare expenditures. These costs are highly concentrated within small segments of the population, with 5 percent of patients associated with more than half of all healthcare dollars spent.[198] When only slightly more than half of all chronic disease patients receive recommended preventive care measures, significant room for improvement exists. This not only justifies the need for better monitoring and management of health, but it likewise demands it.

Given these figures, one effective way to enhance care continuity, care coordination, and patient adherence is through remote monitoring and management solutions. Such solutions offer the means to manage

197   Ibid.
198   Partnership to Fight Chronic Disease, 2016.

patient care outside the physician office or hospital. This may include at-home monitoring and management, or it may involve on-the-go care through mobile devices and other real-time platforms. Through these strategies, continuity of care extends across the entire spectrum of patient activities both within the healthcare system and outside of it. Data and information from one point is shared to the next, and as a result, costs are reduced, compliance enhanced, and quality of patient outcomes improved.

Given the potential of remote monitoring and management solutions, not surprisingly this sector is expected to grow significantly in the coming years. Current estimates suggest remote care platforms will expand by 13 percent by the year 2020, and annual growth is expected to reach nearly 50 percent on average for the next five years. This growth is already evident with remote monitoring and management offerings doubling since 2015. In fact, many hospitals are beginning to utilize these solutions to enhance operational efficiencies, control costs, improve quality of care, and develop more effective risk-management strategies.[199]

In addition to the HRRP and the rise in chronic disease rates expected, other factors also encourage the use of remote health management solutions. Overall, a shift from volume-based healthcare to value-based healthcare will incentivize strategies that seek to reduce complications, promote patient safety, and enhance quality. A major part of this shift will include involvement of patients in their own self-care along with greater transparency of healthcare information and patient accountability. Physician shortages will also promote use of such solutions and patient self-care, as reduced healthcare resources will require alternatives. And the increasing use of mobile devices and telehealth platforms will facilitate remote care approaches, suggesting

---

199   Dan Bowman, "Steady growth for remote patient monitoring market predicted through 2020," *Fierce Healthcare*, 2015, http://www.fiercehealthcare.com/it/steady-growth-for-remote-patient-monitoring-market-predicted-through-2020.

this is both a viable and efficient means to address the many issues facing healthcare today.

Challenges to remote health management will remain to be solved. With any HIT solution, and especially those with external connectivity outside a hospital or healthcare office, privacy and security concerns over patient data are present. Likewise, the cost of some HIT solutions can be a deterrent, as has been seen with EHR in years past. Other challenges include regulations and healthcare policies that lag behind technological advancement. And a continued lack of a standardized reimbursement model for using such solutions can also be problematic. Any remote monitoring and management system must address these key areas in order to be attractive and effective.

Human and Artificial Intelligence

The current US healthcare system has developed based primarily on an acute care model of healthcare services. Because hospital systems have historically provided services and were designed to address disease treatment, a hierarchical model was designed involving a variety of healthcare professionals. This model can be best described as vertical, or at least quasi-vertical, consisting of various levels of medical expertise. For example, different allied health professionals provide lower-level services, with physicians occupying higher levels. This model is less collaborative in nature and more sequential in its functioning, as information flows up or down as services are rendered.

To demonstrate this model in a hospital context, nurses and nursing assistants may provide information regarding vital signs, medication reactions, and other patient-level data to physician assistants, nurse practitioners, or physicians. Some routine services may then be addressed by physician assistants or nurse practitioners, but in more complex instances, information continues upward to physicians and specialists. Once information reaches the designated level where it can be processed, analyzed, and interpreted, instructions for subsequent patient services then flow back downward. Nurses, nursing assistants, or other allied health providers then carry out these instructions. This reflects the classic model of acute healthcare.

Newer models of care are being adopted today in different settings to highlight the need for more collaborative care. For several years, rehabilitative settings have pursued more of a horizontal or team approach to healthcare services. In this model, an array of healthcare professionals, including physicians and allied health providers, communicate and exchange ideas as a means to formulate a collaborative care plan for patients. This model is being increasingly adopted in other hospital settings as well, including dialysis centers, stroke units, and others. These collaborative models have demonstrated enhancements in patient care outcomes while also reducing medical errors, omissions, and waste. In addition, a collaborative model offers greater opportunities for prevention and health promotion for patients through combined expertise and provider education.

Unfortunately, effective collaborative models of care have yet to develop well in outpatient settings. Inherent fragmentation of services results in an inability for all care providers to communicate efficiently, share information, and formulate a cohesive plan. In addition, physicians are typically responsible for overseeing this coordination of care for their patients, and the system hinders them from effectively accomplishing these tasks. Unlike hospitals, nursing homes, and other healthcare facilities, outpatient services lack a physical location where multiple healthcare services can coordinate care. Likewise, care requests are typically left up to the patient and/or caregiver to initiate. Once again, this creates a "reactive" situation rather than a preventive or health promotion environment.

The US healthcare system is primarily dependent upon human intelligence. In acute, collaborative, and outpatient models of care, services are analyzed and determined through various levels of human knowledge and expertise. Each physician and healthcare professional offers knowledge inputs in different situations to best guide patient care. While some of these models are more efficient and thorough in gathering this human intelligence to direct healthcare, all utilize a tremendous amount of human resources in doing so. This is one of the reasons that human resource costs in healthcare are by far the largest expenditure, as one in every eight Americans are employed within this sector.[200]

While human intelligence is essential to an effective healthcare system, HIT solutions offer the use of other forms of intelligence that can enhance efficiency, improve quality, and reduce errors. Artificial intelligence (AI), by definition, refers to the ability of some type of information technology to independently perform cognitive activities that would otherwise be expected to be performed by a human brain. In addition to having an ability to acquire and store knowledge, AI also performs functions related to judgment and understanding as well the capacity to originate new thoughts. Because of this ability, AI could potentially replace human intelligence within healthcare settings, thus reducing human resource demands.[201]

In addition to human resource benefits, AI offers additional advantages as well. For one, once AI is developed, the ability to reproduce these functions is expedited with near infinite potential. Second, since AI devices do not require sleep, extended access to both volume and duration of intelligence could be gained. However, the current state of development of AI has not reached a level where this is a complete reality. AI systems are unable to identify when a problem lacks a solution. Likewise, AI malfunctions can lead to wrong solutions,

---

200   All things considered, "US healthcare workforce larger than ever," *NPR*, 2012, http://www.npr.org/2012/03/19/148939366/u-s-health-care-workforce-larger-than-ever.

201   Jatin Borana, "Applications of artificial intelligence & associated technologies," *Science Proceeding of International Conference on Emerging Technologies in Engineering, Biomedical, Management and Science, March 5–6*, 2016.

which could have significantly negative consequences.[202] While AI represents great potential in healthcare for the future, continued evolution and progress is needed to realize its full potential.

Expert Machine Systems

Though AI is still developing, this does not preclude the use of many of its IT qualities within a healthcare setting. Expert machine systems are routinely used in many areas of healthcare today, and their potential for expanded use is growing exponentially. In essence, expert systems contain extensive expertise within a specific area of interest. Through the use of statistical analysis and data mining, these systems are able to use deductive logic to arrive at solutions and/or recommendations. Once an expert system is constructed with its necessary components, it is then capable of providing extensive analyses which can guide healthcare services more effectively and efficiently.[203]

Expert machine systems have essentially three required components. The first component involves a knowledge base, which contains information, data, and their interrelationships regarding a special area of interest. This knowledge is stored for access, retrieval, and processing. The second component then includes some type of inference engine. When an expert system is queried, this component searches the knowledge base, analyzes its findings, and then responds with a solution or recommendation for the query. Last, an expert system contains a rule component, which is able to relate specific conditions used to develop the solution or recommendation.

Within healthcare today, expert systems are utilized in many areas. One common use is within alert and reminder systems regarding patient data. For example, if an expert system is connected to a patient monitor of any type, it can detect specific changes within defined

---

202   Ibid.
203   Ibid.

parameters and produce a visual and/or auditory warning for a provider. Likewise, such systems can also scan test results and diagnostic orders periodically on the patient in order to monitor for aberrant results and provide reminders for comprehensive care, respectively.[204] Such systems are even used in radiology settings for image recognition and interpretation. Some can provide automatic interpretations of images, which can be beneficial for mass screening exams and to assist in bringing potentially abnormal findings for more detailed radiological review.[205] Notably, these uses offer more thorough and higher quality patient care while saving physician resources.

Some inherent difficulties exist when using expert machine systems for radiological images. First, radiological reports are collected in free text, and the natural complexities and ambiguities in describing images via text make it challenging to define rules and algorithms within expert systems. However, ways around these challenges are being developed as we speak. For example, some corporations like IBM have secured massive databases of radiological images. These corporations plan to link these images with patient EHRs and other data sources as a means to develop improved image recognition with patient health conditions and profiles.[206] Eventually, this could result in machine-assisted diagnosis that has greater quality, reduced errors, and marked improvements in efficiency.

Other uses for expert systems within healthcare also exist. Naturally, such systems can serve as retrieval agents and search tools that seek specific information based on a user's preferences and needs. By having an internal knowledge base, knowledge applications can be applied to searches allowing greater data interpretations. As a result,

---

204   Rajendra Akerkar, *Introduction to Artificial Intelligence*, PHI Learning Pvt. Ltd., 2014.

205   Saeed Hassanpour and Curtis P. Langlotz, "Information extraction from multi-institutional radiology reports," *Artificial Intelligence in Medicine* 66 (2016): 29–39.

206   Rovert McMillan and Elizabeth Dwoskin, "IBM crafts a role for artificial intelligence in medicine," *Wall Street Journal*, 2015, http://www.wsj.com/articles/ibm-crafts-a-role-for-artificial-intelligence-in-medicine-1439265840.

a more detailed and refined list of results can be found based on levels of relevance and importance. Other key areas of use involve diagnosis determinations. In rare or complex cases, expert systems can assist in formulating differential diagnostic possibilities with probability rankings. They can also facilitate education for inexperienced providers and medical students.[207]

Perhaps one of the most beneficial areas where expert systems can be utilized involves treatment planning. For existing treatment plans, these systems can scan for various inconsistencies, errors, and omissions and alert physicians and providers to review specific aspects of the plan. At the same time, expert systems can be used to formulate plans based on patient data and existing information. Aligning these interpretations with standardized guidelines established through evidence-based research can achieve greater consistency and thoroughness.[208] Likewise, this once again saves the physician time and energy while also providing a means for ongoing education, feedback, and quality improvement.

Recent advances in genomics similarly offer great opportunities for artificial intelligence and expert machine systems. With the human genomic mapping project, massive amounts of genetic information have been acquired. Likewise, phenotypic profiles of patients related to various genetic combinations are also being increasingly defined. Aggregate data from these sources have the potential to greatly enhance diagnostic and therapeutic capabilities. For example, a patient with a known genetic profile can have their health risks better characterized, which in turn can guide prevention and health promotion efforts more effectively. This can even identify which medications and treatments may be more effective in a particular individual as well.[209]

207   Akerkar, 2014.
208   Ibid.
209   Gillian Bartlett, Vaso Rahimzadeh, Cristina Longo, Lori A. Orlando, Martin Dawes, Jean

In applying expert systems to areas of genomics, large pools of data can begin to predict and identify patterns that would align genetic profiles with phenotypic presentations. As a result, such systems could screen patient data and clinical profiles as a means to predict how their unique genetic makeup may present in a clinical situation later in life. These same pools of data would then be used to analyze the correlation between genetics, phenotypes, and response to different treatments. Ultimately, this would help construct a large database of information which could be quickly accessed to aid in constructing diagnostic possibilities and optimal treatment options.[210]

Data mining and information extraction offer tremendous potential for the future of healthcare. As global health systems become interconnected over time, this potential expands to an even greater degree. The ability to perform better disease surveillance, gain real-time decision supports, and have access to content-based imaging data will continually facilitate the use of expert systems (and more highly developed artificial intelligence) to guide healthcare more effectively while simultaneously utilizing existing resources more favorably.[211] But even today, many of these advantages are being realized.

Despite these multiple areas where expert systems may be beneficial, they remain significantly underutilized in today's healthcare environment for several reasons. First, expert systems require sufficient data input to be effective. Unfortunately, various EHR systems and other digital sources of healthcare data fail to communicate adequate inputs for expert systems to be fully effective. Second, many expert systems have poor user interface designs. As a result, the inefficiencies and frustrations deter physicians and other providers from their use.[212] This combined with workflow interruptions can serve as barriers to use.

Lachaine, Murielle Bochud, et al., "The future of genomic testing in primary care: the changing face of personalized medicine," *Personalized Medicine* 11, no. 5 (2014): 477–486.
210   Ibid.
211   Hassanpour, 2016.
212   Akerkar, 2014.

Fortunately, innovative solutions are being developed to overcome these barriers. A number of artificial intelligence systems are being implemented in various health centers around the world. For example, some systems are being used to track the evolution and spread of specific pathogens in relation to hospital-acquired infections. Others are being utilized to monitor patients' sleep remotely with concurrent analysis, and some have developed personalized treatment plans based on lifestyle data and patient history. Others are involved in health monitoring activities. For example, some systems are using facial recognition and tracking to monitor medical compliance, and others provide continual patient reminders for testing and treatment. And even administratively, AI systems are facilitating scheduling of services based on patient census, staffing, levels of acuity, and historical trends data.[213] Given these advances, expert systems and AI will clearly be the future of healthcare, and to some extent, this future has already arrived.

ikioo Remote Health Monitoring and Management

In keeping with the concepts discussed thus far, ikioo Remote Health Monitoring and Management offers an innovative artificial intelligence platform to facilitate bringing healthcare into the twenty-first century. In essence, ikioo provides a "health-bot" capable of operating twenty-four hours a day, seven days a week to provide a setting where providers and patients can interact in any environment. While such interactions and coordination of care have primarily existed within hospitals and other healthcare facilities, ikioo enables these same interactions to occur in outpatient areas of care. This not only includes physician offices but likewise home settings, pharmacies, diagnostic

---

213   Bruce, Anne, and Dolly Hinshaw, "Perspective in the acute care continuum," *CEP America*, 2015, http://www.cepamerica.com/news-resources/perspectives-on-the-acute-care-continuum/2015-december/most-popular-2-artificial-intelligence.

centers, and other care areas. In fact, ikioo offers the same opportunities in any location at any time providing an on-the-go forum for healthcare coordination.

The ikioo Remote Health Monitoring and Management system is a software application and hardware platform used by patients and consumers to connect and interact with physicians and other healthcare providers. At the same time, the platform operates a provider portal through which healthcare professionals enjoy access to patient data and information. The application utilizes embedded AI in conjunction with individuals' PHRs to better coordinate care, to connect patient and physician, and to enhance care efficiencies. And in the process, quality of care and patient safety increases.

As the name implies, the ikioo platform consists of both monitoring and management components. The monitoring component allows physicians and providers to evaluate a number of patient attributes and behaviors in a real-time fashion. By defining preset time intervals, which may range from monthly to continuous, providers can determine sets of objective data they wish to monitor. Rules and values are defined that serve as guides for the platform to trigger notifications and alerts to physicians and the entire care team depending on who might need to be informed of the change. In addition, additional information can be accessed at that point to determine additional situational variables and contexts that may affect patient data values.

As an example of ikioo monitoring platform functions, a physician who prescribes a new blood pressure medication for a patient in the office can then assess its response subsequently at any time using the provider portal. As the patient provides additional data regarding blood pressure measurements, through other providers' measurements or through their own measurements, the data is entered into the patient's PHR as part of the ikioo platform. If the values exceed specific defined triggers, the physician is notified. Unlike previous home and mobile situations where such data was unavailable, the ikioo platform allows real-time connection to this objective data. No longer does the physician and other provider have to rely on subjective input from patients and caregivers. Instead, objective measurements and data from other providers and from patients' self-monitoring become instantaneously available.

The monitoring component of the ikioo system has numerous potential uses and advantages. In addition to evaluating treatment responses, the same monitoring can provide information about medication and treatment adherence. Likewise, monitoring functions can be set to identify early diagnosis triggers, which could prompt earlier evaluations for better care. And a variety of patient lifestyle aspects could be monitored, including dietary choices, exercise and activity levels, sleep duration and quality, and stress responses. Each of these monitoring opportunities serve to offer a more comprehensive care environment to patients when outside the hospital and physician's office. And it links all providers on a patient's care team by having access to the same real-time information.

The second component of the ikioo Health Remote Monitoring and Management platform consists of enhanced patient management. With greater data access and notifications determined by patient triggers, the opportunity to provide better management decisions for patient care also exists. Currently, many management decisions rely on patient and caregiver self-reports over the phone or in the office. Likewise, one provider may have information that prompts a care decision that other providers may lack. The result is a disjointed, fragmented management process with multiple "cooks in the kitchen" operating independently in many circumstances to determine patient management. In contrast, using the ikioo platform, the opportunity to collaborative and have coordinated care decisions for a patient is present.

Let's take the same example of the patient requiring blood pressure medication. In a traditional outpatient setting, a family physician prescribes a diuretic for the patient. The patient begins taking the medication, but fails to relay this change in medications to his or her occupational therapist. The patient's occupational therapist has been working with the patient on toileting activities at home due to severe arthritis. Over the course of the next week, the increase in urinary frequency results in the patient falling on the way to the bathroom and sustaining a hip fracture. The lack of care coordination in this instance may not be directly related to the injury, but had the diuretic information been available to the entire care team, alternative choices might have been made. The physician might have chosen a different blood pressure medication, or the occupational therapist might have taken additional safety measures.

This example highlights how better coordination and continuity of care supports better management decisions. At the same time, the ikioo platform also allows physicians to personalize management decisions in alignment with a specific individual patient. Increasingly, many patients do not respond to treatments precisely as planned or may have unexpected results from a treatment. By having access to real-time patient data, the opportunity to tailor treatment to the individual's specific response becomes increasingly possible. Greater knowledge of dietary factors, lifestyle factors, and other specific information can offer a chance to adjust therapies for better personalized care. By linking PHRs with other health information and AI, physicians can manage patients as unique individuals to a better extent rather than lumping all patients with a single disease into one catch-all category.

ikioo Remote Health Monitoring and Management platform also helps physicians through AI-backed clinical decision supports. Equipped with patient and provider data, more comprehensive information can be used to help clinicians determine the best course of action. In addition, standards and clinical guidelines related to specific patient aspects and values can be identified, further guiding better care. And as information is acquired from individual and collective responses to care, these same guidelines can be refined and improved. Each of the management areas is enhanced through the ikioo platform, leading to enhanced patient safety and quality of care. And all of this is possible regardless of a patient's location . . . whether at home or on the go.

The ikioo Remote Health Monitoring and Management platform can be utilized across multiple devices, operating systems, and platforms using standard HL7 language guidelines, thus enabling all healthcare stakeholders to connect and facilitate care coordination. This solution is ideal for chronic disease management outside hospital environments, but at the same time, it can also be utilized for acute care situations as well. In essence, the ikioo platform offers an innovative solution for today's fragmented healthcare environment, and it once again permits physicians and patients to connect in a way that is meaningful and rewarding while providing optimal care.

Summary Considerations

The US healthcare system is fraught with problems. With multiple providers and stakeholders, the system is disjointed with a lack of effective care coordination. Likewise, historical trends have resulted in a focus on acute care management at the expense of prevention and health promotion. And volume, fee-for-service patterns remain despite a changing regulatory landscape. As a result, our healthcare system is fragmented, inefficient, costly, and at times ineffective.

While this description of healthcare services in the US pertains to all settings of care, the most significantly affected environment is outpatient care. Such settings do not provide strong environments for care coordination among various providers, and the ability to maintain a strong patient-physician relationship is challenging at best. With the increase in chronic disease occurrence, and with shifts toward higher volumes of outpatient care services, solutions that address these issues are needed. In addition to enhancing care coordination and information sharing, such solutions need to also personalize healthcare services so optimal care is aligned with patient response. This nuanced care has the opportunity to reduce costs, improve outcomes, and enhance patient safety.

The use of HITs can provide such solutions. Specifically, artificial intelligence and expert machine systems can facilitate knowledge sharing, clinical guideline development, individualized care, and many other areas of healthcare. In addition, such systems allow an extension for coordinated care in various settings including at-home and on-the-go. The ikioo Remote Health Monitoring and Management system utilizes such technologies to provide physicians and patients with the enhanced means to evaluate, assess, and care for various health conditions. As a result, the ikioo system reflects an innovative and creative solution for twenty-first-century healthcare.

While artificial intelligence and expert machine systems provide many advantages in healthcare, these naturally do not eliminate the need for human intelligence as well. Human intelligence and oversight will always be a necessity for healthcare. However, by combining human with artificial intelligence, efficiencies can be gained, quality of care improved, and resource utilization enhanced. Given the focus on value, quality, and efficiency of healthcare services in the twenty-first century, the ikioo Remote Monitoring and Management platform offers physicians a way to pursue these goals while still focusing on optimal patient care and relations.

CHAPTER 7

ikioo Technologies, Inc.
Twenty-First-Century Vision

Given the challenges and pressures of twenty-first-century healthcare, a number of key areas require new directions of change. Each of these areas is not necessarily a stand-alone issue since they all work in concert to bring about innovative change that achieve quality and value goals. However, each may be considered separately as a means to better understand needed areas of change compared to the current healthcare system approach. At the same time, each point of vision can be evaluated in relation to ongoing regulatory and social change.

Expanding Provider Scope of Services

A major point for future change involves the ability to expand the scope of provider services. This naturally involves physician healthcare services, but also includes allied health and other healthcare professional services as well. Despite emphasis being placed on prevention and health promotion, the healthcare system continues to have institutions that focus on reactive medicine addressing illness and disease. This perspective limits the ability of healthcare providers to make substantial impacts on population health, and it hinders effective management of chronic disease. The scope of provider effects must expand in order to meet key healthcare objectives for the future.

From a foundational perspective, medical and allied health teaching curriculums need to better reflect the needs of the healthcare system. While the applied medical sciences are important for understanding both health and pathologic states, their application to clinical practice of healthcare needs to be reconsidered. Instead of applying this knowledge to disease and illness management alone, prevention and health promotion strategies need to represent a heightened component of these curriculums. Lifestyle and dietary choices by patients alone result in substantial impacts of population health and healthcare service utilization, and educating providers in how best to influence these choices is critical for advancing healthcare quality.

At the same time, such curriculums and training opportunities must assist providers in better practice management skills. Based on shifts in reimbursement rates with attention to quality outcomes and performance metrics, providers who best understand how to shift inputs, control costs, and gain optimal outcomes will be most likely to succeed. This is also important in attaining healthcare objectives, as it helps ensure greater sustainability among provider practices over time. In contrast, inability to address these measures could result in costs exceeding reimbursements and subsequent practice failures. This would not only be detrimental to individual provider practices but also to the system as a whole, given the presence of provider shortages.

Last, expansion of providers' scope of healthcare services should involve greater interactions among various healthcare providers. Collaborative models of care in both inpatient and outpatient settings have demonstrated this approach offers better comprehensive care to patients while also allowing a broader array of expertise for patients to access. Collaborative care results in better use of resources, better information sharing, and better clinical outcomes. Adopting models, technologies, and systems that foster and support collaboration among healthcare providers, particularly outside of healthcare facilities, will be essential for the future of healthcare.

"Away from Hospital" Resource Allocation

Based on recent data, roughly two-thirds of every healthcare dollar in the US is spent in outpatient settings outside of hospitals and skilled nursing facilities. While some of these dollars reflect office-based care, many healthcare services also involve community healthcare services and homecare services. Even so, resources are concentrated more heavily in inpatient settings, and the ability to enhance resource utilization in home settings in particular is limited. This reflects an area that needs to change in the future in order to promote better population health. With shifts toward chronic disease monitoring and management, outpatient services, and self-care, it only makes sense to pursue the ability to utilize resources in these settings.

Even within office-based settings and many home settings, traditional face-to-face care remains the norm. But once a patient leaves a physician's office, or after a healthcare provider leaves the patient's home, healthcare services are still required. Prevention efforts, patient education, health promotion guidance, and disease monitoring are all areas that demand nontraditional services that are typically face-to-face. And while telehealth has been identified by CMS as a face-to-face interaction, it still is underutilized and poorly reimbursed. Through greater investments in nontraditional, away-from-the-hospital care, quality and value of healthcare services can be substantially increased.

In this regard, the ikioo platform offers an ideal solution for such investments. The platform creates a virtual environment where information exchange can occur among numerous healthcare stakeholders, including patients, physicians, and allied health providers. As a result, providers can better collaborate in the monitoring and management of individuals in any setting outside the hospital and office. This, in turn, enables a patient-centric model of care that is both scalable and responsive to patient needs. Likewise, it awards the opportunity to engage patients more frequently so they make better lifestyle choices. Future strategies need to embrace such technologies as a means to achieve better healthcare goals.

Extending Standards of Care to All Patient Settings

Over time, healthcare has adopted standards of care that have primarily evolved through research, clinical knowledge, and provider experiences. However, like other aspects of healthcare, these standards focus on disease management and acute care more than prevention, health promotion, and chronic disease management. Only in the last decade or so have clinical guidelines and best practices based on evidence been advanced to address these other areas. But to date, these standards are still limited due to paucity of research and experience in this mode of healthcare.

Through the use of HITs, AI, and human intelligence, standards of healthcare are rapidly advancing today. In the future, big data and aggregate data analysis will enhance these standards and best practice guidelines. But in addition to these pursuits, healthcare standards must be developed for both mobile and at-home care settings. These reflect new areas of care where standards are clearly lacking, and they involve a greater focus on prevention, monitoring, and health promotion. They also involve an increasing role for patients in their own self-care, which is not a strong component in hospital and office-based environments. With shifts in the scope and focus of healthcare, these standards will need to be developed in order to promote quality and safety.

While these standards will be important, equally important will be developing guidelines for adjusting standards in an effort to provide personalized healthcare to individuals. Nuanced care will become increasingly important as unique, individualized responses to healthcare interventions are realized. While standards will represent a generic guide to patient care and management, tailoring healthcare services to individuals based on genomic data, individual responses, and other variables will be needed. Standards tailored in favor of these pursuits will reflect another area where future healthcare guidelines will be necessary.

Adoption of Health-Centric Health System

The US healthcare system that is focused on disease and illness treatment and diagnosis remains a "reactionary" model of care. As a result, healthcare services are utilized after a condition has developed, and this typically results in the use of greater services at higher costs. Likewise, this undermines overall quality of life for patients since, by definition, patients have suffered the effects of an illness for at least some period of time before care is offered.

In contrast, a health-centric model of care seeks to prevent illness and disease before a condition can develop, and therefore focuses on preserving and maintaining health. In addition, early detection of disease is also part of this model to provide care services to individuals early in a disease course, often before symptoms may have appeared. These strategies utilize fewer resources, lower healthcare costs, and improve quality of care and life. Given the excessive expenditures of the US healthcare system, this model is not only desirable but essential.

To help support a health-centric model of care, the ACA has invoked several measures to encourage a shift in this direction. These incentives and requirements can be categorized according to gender and age, as different prevention, screening, and health promotion services are required for different groups. The most generalized group pertains to all adults. For example, within ACA requirements, alcohol abuse, depression, high blood pressure, obesity, and tobacco use screening is mandatory for all adults. Likewise, dietary and sexually transmitted disease education and counseling is required, as is a variety of age-appropriate immunizations. And for high-risk or age-specific populations, abdominal aortic aneurysm, cholesterol, colorectal cancer, type 2 diabetes mellitus, HIV, and syphilis evaluations are included. The ACA requires all health insurance providers to offer these services without any copay, co-insurance, or deductible costs to patients as long as the services are provided by an in-network provider.

For women, the ACA requires insurers to provide an even greater number of preventive and health-promoting services. For example, anemia, bacteriuria, tobacco use, and domestic violence screening is required for all women, while education, counseling, and support for breastfeeding, contraception use, breast cancer genetic risks, and well-women evaluations are also included. For women with specific risk factors and/or age ranges, additional screening and testing must also be provided for various sexually transmitted diseases, human papilloma virus, osteoporosis, cervical cancer, breast cancer, and gestational diabetes mellitus. Last, women who are pregnant must have access to folic acid supplementation, and for specific-risk women, breast cancer chemoprevention must be provided.

Children and adolescents must be screened for alcohol and drug use, behavioral issues, developmental issues, obesity, anemia, and vision disorder screenings. Likewise, children and teens with specific age or behavioral risks are screened for autism, cervical dysplasia, depression, hypothyroidism, dyslipidemia, hearing impairment, sickle cell disease, HIV infection, lead exposure, oral health problems, phenylketonuria, and tuberculosis. Required health promotion services for this age group include fluoride chemoprevention, newborn gonorrhea ocular treatments, age-specific immunizations, and iron supplementation for newborns. And for teens, support and education are to be provided regarding sexually transmitted diseases.

It is evident that part of the focus of the ACA has been to move toward greater prevention and health promotion as a means to improve the quality, value, and efficiency of the US healthcare system. This makes logical sense, and additional measures that adopt a more health-centric model will be part of any effective strategy in the twenty-first century. We should embrace utilization of technologies that facilitate this shift since these will well align with anticipated needs for effective population health.

Establish Early Diagnosis Triggers

As part of developing better standards and guidelines for healthcare services, and along with an effort to design a more personalized, nuanced care model, the advancement of early diagnosis triggers will be important as well. Screening measures may be ineffective if not combined with the ability to formulate accurate and timely diagnoses for management. Therefore, advancing a system that uses data and information to efficiently identify conditions as early as possible becomes important.

The presence of many acute illness triggers can certainly be combined with screening services to augment early disease detection. But this same area for chronic disease detection can be greatly enhanced through better data and information management. For example, the use of family history data and genomics for individual patients can be used to not only identify risk but to look for the presence of early disease since knowledge of this information can result in more aggressive screening measures. While some of this has occurred within healthcare currently, this area has great potential for expansion, leading to better healthcare.

Utilizing technologies to assist in these efforts and to guide early diagnosis detection offers a tremendous opportunity to enhance healthcare services. The ikioo Health Monitoring and Management system utilizes AI software to assess collected data from screenings while applying this data to known guidelines and standards. As increasing data collection and analysis permits advancement of these parameters, earlier detection of conditions becomes increasingly possible. As a result, screening efforts become more effective and care becomes more personalized.

Developing a Comprehensive Milieu of Care

In the twenty-first century, not only will care shift from a disease-centric model to a health-centric one, but care will also become more patient centric and decentralized. Increased mobility, diversity of service settings, and on-demand service is the norm as information technologies have advanced. The same will occur within healthcare as consumers increasingly demand such changes in an effort to gain the care they want. As a result, a more comprehensive milieu of care will be needed to expand the setting, timing, and drivers of healthcare provisions.

Four main cornerstones underlie the development of such a milieu. The first cornerstone involves the decentralization of care services. Under current models, physicians provide more of a centralized source where allied health providers and patients receive instructions and guidance in a vertical structure model. This model will need to change for services to become more patient centric and to allow better utilization of resources. This does not imply that physicians, and in particular the physician-patient relationship, will be any less important; however, greater access to care services, collaboration among various providers, and enhanced transparency of information will create a more horizontal structure where care can be enhanced at lower costs.

The next cornerstone of this milieu of care services will involve greater mobility of data. Notably, data is highly mobile today in other sectors as mobile devices, software platforms, and information technologies facilitate access from nearly any location. Though healthcare must deal with security and privacy issues to a greater extent, data mobility must be developed in order for decentralization to occur and for healthcare knowledge to be advanced. Platforms, such as ikioo systems, that facilitate data sharing and provider collaboration through secure, protected interfaces will be an essential component in increasing data mobility.

The last two cornerstones needed for developing a more comprehensive milieu of care include measures for on-demand care and home-based care services. Rather than employing care services in an arbitrary manner based on provider schedules and locations, patients and consumers will require more continuous care delivery systems. In other words, healthcare services will be increasingly expected when and where patients want them. From an on-demand perspective, enhanced transparency of information and data will be needed, in addition to improved patient-provider communications. In terms of home-based care, enhanced patient monitoring and management remotely will be needed. These facets will have dramatic impacts on the US healthcare system and will greatly improve care service quality.

Moving from the current model of care to a more comprehensive system will not occur overnight. Stepwise movement in this direction should occur, however, with the eventual goal of delivering seamless, continuous care to patients in a real-time, mobile, on-demand fashion. The ikioo system promotes this type of strategy with progressive movement from monthly to weekly to progressively shorter care intervals until continuous monitoring and management care is realized. Having a system in place that permits evolution into a continuous care model is essential to achieve a comprehensive care milieu.

Embedded AI Software Assistance

Over the last few decades, the expansion of information has been exponential. This fact is certainly relevant to healthcare in several areas, with genomics being one of the most exciting areas, among many. But with this expansion, the ability for any one person or entity to maintain high levels of expertise in numerous fields has been extremely difficult if not impossible. Utilizing technology to assist with these challenges makes perfect sense, to optimize healthcare quality without increasing costs.

Embedding AI software into various healthcare systems provides an array of opportunities for enhanced healthcare. As discussed previously, the use of EHR is limited by vendors and their ability to readily transfer patient information from one provider to the next. PHRs offer additional health data and information, but integration of EHR systems with PHRs is rather poor in today's healthcare market. Embedded AI platforms offer the chance to provide greater data transferability and EHR-PHR integration to remedy these problems. Specifically, the ikioo Health Monitoring and Management system enables consolidation of systems in one virtual location for better access and data retrieval.

By utilizing AI software, healthcare systems and providers can move away from having to track down patient data from various sources. Instead, patient data will follow the patient to any point in the healthcare system, an efficient system that allows much improved communication among patients and providers. As a result, providers are more likely to be on the same page, patients more likely to understand instructions, and healthcare systems to operate at lower costs and with greater safety outcomes.

In addition to these benefits, embedded AI also facilitates better provider decisions through decision support systems based on established clinical guidelines. Better chronic disease management results through use of alerts, reminders, and triggers utilized to overcome current human errors and system inefficiencies. Also, real-time patient inputs can be entered into data systems, further enabling mobility, on-demand services, and multisetting care. AI systems also permit development of more comprehensive care plans through better information access and provider collaboration. Healthcare in the coming decades can benefit greatly from the use of AI platforms based on these benefits alone.

Use of Predictive Technologies and Analytics

From a larger perspective, healthcare systems must utilize AI as part of predictive technologies and analytics when considering future advances. The progress that has been made in data mining, software applications, big data analytics, and other technologies supports the progressive use of predictive analytics to assist providers with clinical care. Currently, predictive technologies have already been utilized to enhance billing systems, payment processing, and administrative areas such as appointment scheduling. But increasingly, their value in clinical care is being appreciated and realized.

Predictive technologies in essence use structured inputs and data sets from relational databases to identify patterns, associations, and risks associated with subsequent outcomes. In other words, predictive models require inputs as well as feedback regarding the effect of those inputs. For example, a patient may have a dozen specific data inputs regarding various lifestyle factors, which may include tobacco use, high blood pressure, excessive weight, and others. Each of these inputs are then analyzed through predictive models to determine actual risks for developing a specific condition like a heart attack. By pooling thousands upon thousands of patients into these models, increasing accuracy can result, allowing better quality and efficiency of decision making and resource utilization.

Of course, predictive technologies cannot determine calculated risks without receiving continuous feedback regarding outcomes. In order to determine the weight of a specific patient attribute, the association of this attribute with an outcome must be continually refined as increasing datasets become available. Also, predictive technologies use statistical processing to assign various "weights" to these inputs based on their association with an outcome. Then, once all input weights are known, an actual total calculated risk for an outcome can be provided. In the previous example of a heart attack, each of the lifestyle attributes would be assigned a weighted value and then combined to give a provider the actual risk for that patient having a heart attack.

Naturally, if predictive models are well designed and refined, the potential to enhance clinical decision-making efficiency and accuracy is evident. These models will eliminate waste and improve care and patient safety. In addition, resources can be used before disease occurs, thus reducing total resource investments and healthcare costs per patient. The key is to ensure such predictive technologies and models receive the data required and are constantly refined to provide advancing quality decision making and care. Through the use of AI and natural language processing, these goals can be accomplished, and physicians are well situated to serve as champions of these needed healthcare changes.

Health bots can be envisioned to provide such predictive technologies in healthcare settings. Health bots are essentially intelligent systems that interact with end users, providing an array of data analysis and information through the use of AI, natural language processing, and other technologies, including predictive analytics. Bots are designed to provide a more natural interaction with patients and providers, enhancing value in numerous areas. For example, health bots can be used to interact with patients through web portals to provide education, support, counseling, and specific information. Likewise, health bots can integrate EHR data, PHR data, hospital registration information, billing information, and diagnostic reports for enhanced physician decision making.

The ikioo health bot offers these services through a multi-tiered predictive technology platform. By examining patient lifestyle attributes and analyzing them in relation to patient conditions, the ikioo bot provides physicians better knowledge of patient risk ahead of time so that treatments and changes can be implemented. In addition, these same technologies enhance communications among providers while also more fully integrating patient data. As a result, the ikioo health bot embraces the need for predictive technologies in healthcare and offers a cutting-edge platform through which it can be provided both now and well into the future.

Competition for Private Healthcare Expenditures

Despite many countries having government-sponsored healthcare systems, and despite the US healthcare system relying heavily on Medicare, Medicaid, and private health insurers, the amount of out-of-pocket expenditures by patients and consumers for various healthcare services remains substantial. On average, individuals in the US spend over $1,000 on out-of-pocket healthcare expenses, excluding insurance premiums. When premiums are considered, Americans spend nearly $3,500 on average for healthcare out of their own pockets. In comparison, the average per capita spending in Canada, the next lowest nation, was just under $650 per person.[214] Based on these figures, US healthcare expenses are exorbitant, and private healthcare expenditures are a sizable portion of the healthcare market.

Competition for these healthcare dollars will be necessary. Patients will drive healthcare decisions to a greater extent by voting with their dollars. Patient choice for providers and healthcare organizations

---

214   The Commonwealth Fund, "US healthcare from a global perspective," 2015, http://www.commonwealthfund.org/publications/issue-briefs/2015/oct/us-health-care-from-a-global-perspective.

will become a larger part of healthcare decisions, and private health dollars will follow these choices.

Therefore, competing for these funds by developing stronger patient relations, enhancing quality of care, and reducing costs and waste will be necessary in order to succeed in the healthcare arena. Health monitoring and management technologies facilitate these strategies. In addition, increasing competition for global private health dollars will likely occur as medical tourism and remote healthcare service access expand. Technologies including platforms like the ikioo Health Monitoring and Management system provide the tools to help providers position themselves for such competition. Through the use of AI and predictive technologies, providers will need to distinguish themselves as high quality and highly efficient.

Basic Healthcare Technology Provisions for US Households

As healthcare moves to a more patient centric and health-focused model, provisions will need to be made for US households to accommodate these changes. At the present time, healthcare services essentially operate on a conveyor belt type of system where providers often prescribe medications or arrange for medical devices for patients based on generalized guidelines and standards. Yet, once prescribed or arranged, no subsequent objective evaluations occur in terms of treatment response until the patient returns for the next office visit or until complications have already developed. Not only are these practices inefficient due to inherent delays between the initial treatment and needed adjustments, but they also undermine quality of care.

Increasingly, a need for better individualized care will be required. Rather than simply applying generalized standards to large patient populations with a single diagnosis, individuals' treatment and care plans will be devised based on continuous monitoring data. The patient-centric model demands this type of monitoring as well as patient involvement, and ensuring adequate technologies exist in every US household will be essential. Ongoing objective data can then be received by physicians and other providers so they can make near real-time adjustments in treatments to maximize outcomes and effect.

As an example, millions of patients receive prescriptions for high blood pressure control. However, few have home blood pressure monitoring devices to provide their providers with blood pressure response data to that medication over the days and weeks after a medication is begun. As a result, actual assessment of the blood pressure response to the medication may not occur for several weeks. And during this time, side effects, inadequate response, or adverse reactions might occur, affecting both efficiency of care and quality of care while undermining patient safety.

Based on recent statistics, roughly 125 million households exist in the US today. A home blood pressure monitoring device costs approximately $10, so one device for every home would cost a little over $1 billion. We can compare this figure to the net sales for the top medical device and pharmaceutical companies to place this figure in better perspective. The top one hundred medical device companies yield combined net sales of over $130 billion a year, while the top fifteen pharmaceutical companies exceed a combined net sales of over $525 billion.[215] Investing in more effective home-based monitoring devices and systems makes intuitive sense, and this can help significantly reduce costs of healthcare through enhanced efficiency of services.

Summary Considerations

Healthcare in the twenty-first century will require changes from all healthcare stakeholders. Patients will not only demand greater involvement in their care, but they will also provide increasing amounts

---

215   John LaMattina, "Big Pharma But Not Such Big Money," *Forbes*, March 23, 2015, http://www. forbes.com/sites/johnlamattina/2015/03/23/big-pharma-but-not-such-big-money/#7c027ea83189.

of data and have higher levels of accountability in the process. Insurers and payers will likewise need to adjust through utilizing informatics, shifting covered services to preventive and health promotion activities, and learning how to compete for patient dollars. And physicians will need to embrace a new model of care that is highly mobile, on-demand, and patient centric while expanding communication and collaboration with other healthcare providers. While this shift will occur over an extended period of time and require constant refinement, the direction of this change is inevitable.

In order to move in this direction, patients will need a more comprehensive milieu of care. The use of AI and predictive technologies facilitate this transformation of the US healthcare system, and technologies that are mobile, can integrate data, provide analytics, and facilitate individualized care decisions will be the most effective. The ikioo Health Monitoring and Management platform provides just that. With an understanding of the ten key areas of change needed to advance US as well as global healthcare into the twenty-first century, the ikioo system offers a comprehensive tool for physicians to accomplish these goals.

CHAPTER 8

Twenty-First-Century Health Markets

Without question, the US healthcare system is quite unique in its structure and function. Therefore, appreciating how the system might change in order to meet objectives of a twenty-first-century healthcare vision is a worthwhile endeavor. Change is never accomplished without some degree of resistance and challenge, and this certainly pertains to healthcare in the US. Major efforts will be required to achieve defined goals and avoid many of the impending catastrophes that might affect the healthcare market.

The many variables that demand change include excessive healthcare expenditures, the rising prevalence of chronic disease, an aging population, and large segments with poor access to care. But at the same time, there is great opportunity to revamp a dysfunctional healthcare market to promote innovation, efficiency, and high quality care. Approaching the US healthcare market and change from this viewpoint encourages participation and engagement of all stakeholders and allows a reduced resistance to change.

From this positive vantage point, a number of recommendations can enhance the healthcare market moving forward. Each of these recommendations serves to enhance free market competition, the best solution for proper resource allocation, accurate cost and price mechanisms, and equitable supply and demand development. Many of these recommendations involve the expanding use of technologies to facilitate this change while others involve important legislative and regulatory changes to the system itself. Both are essential to the future success of the American healthcare system. As a result, this chapter will seek to address these issues and solutions in an effort to provide a guide for positive change.

Competition and Healthcare

The US economy in most sectors relies on free market competition as a means to provide the highest quality and the lowest price. Consumers equipped with adequate information about a product or service determine how much they are willing to pay. If companies can meet the price desired, then consumer demand matches the ability to supply those goods. And if several companies can do so, then competition allows costs to fall or quality to advance. This is the nature of a free market system where prices and goods are regulated by consumer preferences.

Free market systems have been said to be led by an "invisible hand." Economist Adam Smith strongly supported this notion, and he believed allowing consumer demand and provider supply to self-regulate a market was the optimal way to allocate resources without developing excess surpluses of goods or shortages. In addition, free market competition allows prices to be determined based on these factors, and therefore, expenditures tend to reflect consumer needs and demand without being excessively high or low.[216] The free market system works effectively in many economic sectors in the US.

Unfortunately, this is not the case for the healthcare sector for a number of reasons. The payment structure of the US healthcare system does not easily allow direct competition over prices. Prices for medical services are typically defined through negotiated or mandated payment structures between providers and payers, and as a result, consumer demand often has a minimal influence on the resulting cost

---

216   Adam Smith, *The Invisible Hand*, vol. 44 (UK: Penguin, 2008).

of healthcare services. Prices are based on other variables such as the cost of educating providers, technologies required, and administrative expenses, and because of this, prices may remain high even if consumer demand falls. This not only results in higher prices but likewise reduced access to care in many instances since some consumers may be unable to afford basic levels of coverage.

In addition to a lack of price flexibility based on consumer demand, healthcare competition is also limited due to a lack of information access. First, consumers generally lack information about the quality of the services they are receiving. While provider report cards are being increasingly utilized, the ability to determine the quality of one provider over another can be challenging at best. This is further hindered by the fact that consumers lack expertise and knowledge about many medical and health conditions when compared to providers. Though the Internet has helped, tremendous gaps in information between providers and consumers continue to exist, resulting in a "blind" reliance on providers. These gaps undermine a competitive environment and can lead to instances of deception, fraud, and excessive costs.

Many other aspects of healthcare pricing further complicate transparency of costs versus pricing. In some instances, healthcare organizations utilize bulk purchasing strategies in an effort to reduce costs through economies of scale. But while some entities are able to pursue this strategy, others cannot. And since the healthcare sector fails to operate in a free market system, cost savings from bulk purchases may not be passed along to consumers. Instead, cost savings are used to augment areas where costs are excessive. This strategy is referred to as cost shifting, and it is routinely employed in healthcare organizational environments.

Another common practice related to healthcare pricing also involves price discriminations. Unlike other sectors which have a single price for all consumers, a healthcare service may be one price for one insurance payer and a different price for another. Since reimbursement schedules are negotiated separately for different payers, a range of reimbursement rates and prices of services are often present. This further complicates the ability to determine the actual cost of a service from a pricing perspective since providers are simply seeking the highest reimbursement regardless of cost. In the absence of competition and a free market, incentives to offer services at the lowest price to cover costs and maintain a competitive profit margin do not exist.

Price discriminations serve to allow healthcare entities the ability to cross-subsidize. In other words, by charging one payer a higher price for a service, additional revenues from this payer are used to subsidize payments received from a payer who is offered lower prices for the same service. The fact that these pricing strategies are allowed further undermines real competition among providers, and it also clouds pricing transparency for consumers. Because prices are typically contractually determined with payers, and because most consumers have a health insurance plan, the opportunity to shop around for the lowest cost health services is not possible. In addition, there is absolutely no incentive to do this since health insurance insulates the consumer from price variations in healthcare services.

The very nature of negotiated and regulated reimbursement rates for healthcare services undermines the ability to replicate a free market environment. Inevitably, some services are reimbursed at higher rates than others, and this determination creates an incentive to provide certain services over those with lower reimbursements. In contrast, free market competition allows the consumer to determine which services are more valuable and in demand rather than a healthcare payer. While reimbursement schedules may attempt to replicate consumer demand, the ability to do so is often impossible due to changing market conditions. As a result, the services often provided may not best fit consumer needs within the US healthcare system.

The use of information technologies has expanded in recent years with electronic medical records, email communications, and electronic prescriptions, but the sharing of information between providers and consumers and among providers remains less than desirable. Between privacy and security concerns and a delay in adopting newer technologies like social media, providers and consumers alike continue to have inadequate information to make fully informed decisions unlike other market sectors of the economy. In order for consumers to make wise decisions about cost versus benefit, this information has to be available.

While reducing price regulations and enhancing information access would aid competition in healthcare greatly, other barriers to competition also exist. For consumers who enjoy some type of health insurance coverage, little incentive exists to discriminate over healthcare services based on cost. This has changed slightly with rising out-of-pocket expenses through copays and deductibles, but still, insurance coverage reduces the tendency for individuals to select a service based on the actual price charged since the deductible or copay does not change. Thus, while other markets are often driven by price, insured individuals do not necessarily feel the need to base decisions on cost in healthcare . . . even if such information is available.

Another obstacle is that a great deal of uncertainty exists when it comes to various diseases and conditions. One person may respond well to a treatment while another person does not. Likewise, predicting if someone may develop a chronic condition over time is incredibly difficult. Therefore, insurers, providers, and consumers all lack a degree of information about outcomes of care. This makes it incredibly challenging for truly competitive environments to develop since the ability to compare one service to another based on patient responses is variable.

Given these issues in healthcare, the ability to allow a competitive, free market to develop has been limited. Regulations in price, gaps in information, uncertainty, and poor incentives plague the system, and each undermines true competition where consumer demand could drive cost efficiency and higher quality of care. Fortunately, some of these areas can be improved while others cannot. But as it stands today, these barriers to competition continue to exist and limit the power that a market economy might have on improving the system overall.

Regulation and Healthcare

Over the course of many decades, an abundance of regulatory oversight has been put into place to govern the healthcare sector. Initially, regulations were established for providers, hospitals, and other aspects of care to ensure high-quality services for society, but as costs and expenditures began to rise, regulations that controlled prices were also invoked. Unfortunately, a system-wide approach was not pursued, and as a result, regulations were implemented haphazardly without paying attention to prior policies.

Lack of integration in developing regulations in the healthcare sector has greatly contributed to its inefficiencies and the lack of competition. Having a government that is both a payer and a regulator causes further problems. Naturally, price regulation ensured cost containment to a degree, but cost was never linked to quality. In addition, because prices were not subject to consumer demand, arbitrarily high prices forced some individuals out of the healthcare market, resulting in increased uninsured populations. And since providers did not have to compete based on quality or price, innovation and advancement in delivering better healthcare became stagnant.

These were not the only negative effects of government regulations in healthcare. Price controls also created perverse incentives. In other words, rather than pursuing quality care for lower cost with the use of fewer resources, no deterrent existed to utilize increasing amounts of resources. This not only satisfied the ethical need for providers to provide higher quality services, but it also reimbursed them higher amounts for a higher volume of services performed. Restrictions on provider training similarly created barriers to entry for competition, as did laws that limited some provider functions. And all the while, administrative and legal costs to ensure regulatory compliance further added costs to the healthcare system.

Repeatedly, central planning efforts in regulating any economy have been shown to be ineffective. The ability to predict consumer preferences is beyond the scope of such efforts, and the complexity of consumer decision making at any given time is nearly impossible to anticipate. As a result, the distribution of resources becomes inequitable, and supply and demand fail to properly align. Perverse incentives further negatively affect the market. Ultimately, surpluses and shortages of healthcare services result in different areas, and access to needed healthcare by some populations is restricted. This is the current state of the US healthcare market due to over-regulation by government policies and legislation.

Potential Solutions to Enhance Healthcare Competition

A number of potential solutions can help overcome lack of competition. Of course, none of the solutions will be as ideal as a free market situation, but changes can be made to better align consumer needs and demands with provider and payer incentives as a means to approximate this ideal situation. Certainly, some changes have helped in this regard including enhanced quality reporting measures and penalties for poor patient outcomes such as re-hospitalization rates and hospital acquired complications. But certainly more needs to be done.

Some solutions are related to the use of advanced technologies while others relate to changes in market regulations and functions. Likewise, others promote greater innovation and involvement of the consumer to better construct a free market type of system.

Increase Healthcare Market Transparency

Transparency can be defined as the intentional sharing of information from a sender to another entity, and involves three key characteristics. The first characteristic involves disclosure. Disclosure relates to the purposeful action of one person or organization to reveal details of an interaction, transaction, or activity. In healthcare, this may pertain to the occurrence of a medical error, an itemization of activities that occurred during a hospital visit, or a number of other events. By disclosing such information, healthcare providers build trust with consumers and other stakeholders, and at the same time empower patients to make better decisions about their care.

The second aspect of transparency involves clarity. Clarity refers to enabling a good understanding of the details of an action by all parties involved. Informed consent laws address this to an extent, requiring providers to ensure patients are clear about the indications, risks, and alternatives to various interventions. But in addition to these measures, clarity can be enhanced by providing education and information in ways that patients can easily comprehend. Clarity fosters patient knowledge and enhances patient engagement, accountability, and participation in the healthcare process.

The third characteristic of transparency pertains to accuracy. A lack of accuracy is often present in various cost centers of healthcare. For example, hospital charges for a single tablet of acetaminophen may cost as much as an entire bottle bought at a pharmacy as an outpatient. Or diagnostic procedures may be markedly increased over the actual costs of the procedures without patient knowledge of the real costs. Revealing the details of specific aspects of care, including costs, will help patients as well as the entire market.

A major direction toward enhancing competition relates to transparency of pricing for healthcare services. As noted, pricing is quite complex, and a number of pricing strategies used by healthcare organizations often cloud the picture further. If some higher-priced services are used to offset losses for lower-priced services, this information should be readily apparent to help with cost determinations and organizational efficiency. Before any efforts can be made to allow consumer selection based on price, greater transparency of the actual price for a service must be available.

In free market systems, price transparency is readily available. First, consumers know what they are paying for a product or service since they directly purchase the goods. In healthcare, however, insurance and government providers buffer patients from this knowledge. The second reason free markets have greater price transparency pertains to competition. When a number of competitors compete in a specific market area, prices typically fall. Once again, this phenomenon is not present in healthcare since prices are often regulated by reimbursement rates determined by government and insurance providers. True competition therefore is unable to affect price.

In order to move toward a more patient-centric model of care, transparency must be markedly improved. Patients should be aware of the actual costs of healthcare services and products, and they should have an adequate understanding of these services in order to make educated decisions about their care. Likewise, healthcare providers should embrace transparency, as it promotes trust and a stronger provider-patient relationship. As a result, adherence improves, and patients become more responsible for their care.

Improve Information Sharing

In 2001, the Nobel Memorial Prize in Economics was awarded to George Akerlof, Michael Spence, and Joseph E. Stiglitz for their analyses of markets with asymmetric information. In contract theory and economics, information asymmetry deals with the study of transaction decisions where one party has more or better information than the other. This creates an imbalance of power in the transaction, which can sometimes cause the transaction to go awry.[217]

Different models involving information asymmetry exist. In adverse selection models, the ignorant party lacks information while negotiating an agreed contract. An example of adverse selection might pertain to a high-risk individual who would be more likely to buy health insurance because the insurance company cannot effectively discriminate against them. This might occur because the insurance company lacks information about that particular individual's risk, or it may result from regulatory constraints.

In contrast, in moral hazard situations, the ignorant party lacks information about performance of the agreed-upon transaction or lacks the ability to retaliate for a breach of the agreement. An example of a moral hazard might involve an individual who behaves recklessly after becoming insured. This might occur because the insurer cannot observe the behavior or effectively retaliate against it. One example might be a person who denies tobacco use yet actually smokes tobacco, or another might be where an insurer can no longer cancel a health insurance policy even if they learn of the tobacco use.

Signaling and screening are two of the primary solutions for this problem. Michael Spence originally proposed the idea of signaling. He proposed that in a situation where information asymmetry exists, it is possible for people to signal their lack of knowledge and thus require the other party to provide the information to resolve the asymmetry. In a healthcare setting, an example of signaling could involve communications between a patient and a health insurer. For a patient who leads a healthy lifestyle, this information could be signaled to an insurer, enabling the patient to receive rewards in insurance premiums as incentives. Alternatively, patients with poor health lifestyles or conditions would similarly signal this information to an insurer.

---

217 Steven Pressman, ed., *Leading Contemporary Economists: Economics at the Cutting Edge* (Routledge, 2008).

However, instead of these patients being denied coverage or having limited care access, government subsidies could be provided that help insurers give greater attention to these individuals. As a result, insurers will want to attract all types of patients since both offer them benefits, and the information sharing provided by signaling facilitates better care, incentivizes healthy lifestyles, and properly allocates healthcare resources.

On the other hand, Joseph E. Stiglitz pioneered the theory of screening. In this situation, the underinformed party induces the other party to reveal their information by providing a menu of choices in such a way that the choice requires use of the private information that the other party has. Tshilidzi Marwala and Evan Hurwitz studied the influence of artificial intelligence on the theory of asymmetric information and observed that artificial intelligence decreases the degree of information asymmetry.[218] Markets where AI is used are thus more efficient by reducing or eliminating information asymmetry.

Certainly, information asymmetry currently exist in the healthcare market today. In addition to needing greater transparency and information about pricing and costs, consumers must also have access to specific information about services and the providers who perform them. To date, provider report cards and performance metrics have been reported in some areas, but research shows that consumers making decisions do not use these resources the majority of the time. Insights into what information consumers want and providing that information in relevant and easy ways for consumers is needed if they are to make logical decisions about their healthcare. Information about service and provider quality is as important as pricing information when trying to approach a situation comparable to a free market environment.

Once pricing and quality data are readily available to consumers, the ability for consumers to make healthcare choices based on this data

---

218	Tshilidzi Marwala and Evan Hurwitz, "Artificial Intelligence and Asymmetric Information Theory," *arXiv preprint arXiv:1510.02867* (2015).

should also be in place. Currently, health insurance coverage insulates consumers from natural incentives to make such choices. Therefore, aligning health insurance coverage to reflect pricing and quality information is needed to encourage consumers to make these decisions more naturally. For example, for higher price services, deductibles and copays would be increased for consumers while those of lower quality and price would be the opposite within their insurance plans. Likewise, services performed by quality performance providers would be incentivized over lower quality providers.

These structures would permit consumers to choose which provider they wanted based on cost and quality, and it would incentivize providers to offer the lowest price possible while offering high quality care. In essence, such a system would utilize various tiers of services based on pricing and quality, and subsequently, consumers could make rational choices within these tiers when given necessary information. As a result, consumer demands would be better aligned with provider services, and while this is not as effective as a free market situation, it is an improvement over the current noncompetitive system.

Adopt Sound Economic Health Screening Models

The difference in information between two agents within healthcare models negatively affects the system as a whole. The agent who has lesser amounts of information seeks to gain information from the other agent. And based on the information gained, different arrangements will be considered as part of a contractual relationship. In healthcare, this situation routinely develops between health insurers and patients, as different insurance coverage packages are offered patients based on the information an insurer has about the patient. If all information is available, then the insurance package best reflects actual costs and services anticipated. But when information asymmetry exists, the package will be inadequate in one way or another. In some situations, costs are excessive and have to be shifted onto other consumers.

By attaining better information symmetry between these agents, better contractual arrangements can be made that serve both parties well in the long run. Patients with poor health and poor lifestyles will require greater services, and therefore cost insurers more. But government assistance can serve to incentivize coverage of these individuals by insurers while also allocating needed resources effectively to a population that needs them. Given the current healthcare model, this does not naturally occur. The resultant information asymmetry hinders effective resource allocation and tends to drive up costs while undermining access and quality.

Effective health screening to target important conditions can help patients achieve major health savings and a significant improvement in quality of life. For example, of the forty-eight million baby boomers receiving Medicare, it is estimated that between one and two million have occult hepatitis C, which may result in major chronic disease costs later in life. But without this knowledge, neither patients nor insurers can negotiate accurate contracts or receive/provide services needed. However, if effective health screening methods were in place, this information could be provided to both parties and facilitate more equitable relationships between the agents.[219]

Naturally, screening for all health conditions is not feasible, as this would also drain resources quickly and undermine the overall objectives of pursuing a better healthcare system. However, the application of economic principles in determining which health screening measures should be performed would help pursue these objectives in a major way. Government involvement in requiring such screenings is important, and these should be implemented so that better prevention and health promotion efforts can be achieved. And at the same time, such health screenings should be pursued as a means to allow greater information symmetry, transparency, and resource allocation.

---

219   CDC, "Why should people born from 1945–1965 get tested for hepatitis C?" 2016, https://www.cdc.gov/knowmorehepatitis/media/pdfs/factsheet-boomers.pdf.

Embed AI in Healthcare Technologies

Embedding AI into healthcare systems and technologies offers improved access to information. In essence, AI has the ability to markedly advance data analysis and pattern recognition, and this can reveal information previously unrecognized by the provider, the patient, and the insurer. This not only has potential at an individual level but also at a population level as risks, treatment response, and other parameters of care can be better identified and addressed.

The use of EHR currently equates to an electronic filing cabinet with poor integration and interconnectivity with other systems. The use of embedded AI has the potential to improve this interoperability. Individual data can then be better combined with public health data, allowing marked advancements in health analytics and health knowledge. Likewise, AI can facilitate better patient safety and reduction of medical errors in a similar manner when embedded into existing HIT systems.

Finally, the use of embedded AI allows a reduction in information asymmetry by providing greater opportunities for signaling and screening. For example, a patient who denies tobacco use yet has nicotine-stained teeth and fingernails can be identified through AI by data discrepancies. This information can then be provided to providers and insurers. Such processes reduce waste, better allocate resources, and reduce costs. In addition, they facilitate a more personalized approach to patient care as greater knowledge of individual genetics and behaviors guide more effective care.

Facilitate Macro and Micro Efficiencies

As a general term, efficiency refers to the ability to achieve a goal through using the least possible resources in the shortest amount of time while maintaining a needed level of quality. This is certainly an ideal objective within healthcare, but the pursuit of economic efficiencies are also important. In this regard, efficiency refers to the ability to change a current economic situation so the welfare of all is improved without reducing the welfare of any particular individual or group. This remains a challenge and a need for healthcare as changes in policies are adopted.

Economic efficiencies in healthcare can be distinguished based on the magnitude of their impact. Macro efficiencies relate to those which affect more than one healthcare market externally. For example, efficiencies that affect both medical device companies as well as health insurers might reflect a macro efficiency. In essence, any change in policy that improves overall welfare between such markets without hindering their function is advantageous for overall healthcare quality. The implementation of CMS bundled payment programs represent an example of a macro efficiency since the consumer receives greater quality of service, providers have opportunities to share in savings, and the insurer (Medicare) reduces their costs.

Micro efficiencies within healthcare refer to those that enhance welfare within individual markets rather than outside of them. In this instance, a policy change results in improvements within a specific healthcare sector without imposing negative effects in the process. An example of this might be recent collaborations among the Drug Enforcement Agency, the Food and Drug Administration, and the Office of National Drug Control Policy to reduce the misuse of opioids and acetaminophen. The collaboration reduced individual resource use and efforts of these agencies while augmenting the overall outcome of their objectives.

In an ideal world, a market would inherently regulate itself as each actor in the market would behave in a rational manner. But such a market does not exist, especially in healthcare. Market actors do not always behave rationally (for example, people choose to smoke despite knowing health risks), and health is not equitably distributed among all individuals. For these reasons, some level of government involvement is needed to ensure welfare, fairness, access, and quality. But this involvement must be aimed at encouraging free market competition and in achieving optimal efficiencies to attain the best level of health welfare.

Maintain Market Equilibriums

In addition to economic efficiencies within and among healthcare markets, market equilibriums are also important to maintain. When markets are in equilibrium, consumer demand equals the supply of healthcare services. As demand shifts and changes, so does supply. In addition, market equilibrium allows for prices to be determined by competition, and the production of services equals the number of services used by patients. This reflects the ideal situation that naturally achieves economic efficiency by reducing surpluses and shortages and by advancing quality and overall welfare through competition.

Unfortunately, the healthcare market and the individuals markets within healthcare are far from ideal. They are not in equilibrium, as supply and demand are not well aligned in many areas, and reimbursements and prices are not based on free market competition. This market disequilibrium results in behaviors among individual healthcare stakeholders that are contrary to optimal efficiency and outcomes. Game theory, which describes a situation where one determines their actions based on the anticipated action of others in a game, has been used to explain this detrimental behavior in markets that are not in equilibrium. In these instances, individuals choose an action that is most likely to advance their own position without concern for others' position in the market.

The recent restriction in medical residency slots offers a perfect example of such behaviors in the healthcare market. In 2016, over 42,000 trained medical school graduates sought residency training positions. However, less than 31,000 slots were made available. In fact, the number of training slots was reduced in response to declining physician reimbursement rates in the market. By restricting residency training slots, and thus future physician numbers, a greater amount of reimbursement dollars would be available per physician. However, this is contrary to market needs. A relative physician shortage exists in primary care currently, and demand for all physician services is expected to increase by 17 percent in the next decade. The restriction of residency training slots demonstrates a behavior that is self-serving but fails to appreciate total market needs.

Healthcare markets are highly interdependent, and in order to avoid detrimental behaviors among individual market actors, market equilibrium between supply and demand is needed. Free market competition facilitates this, but in its absence, government policies need to align incentives to better match supply and demand within and among the various healthcare markets. Maintaining an equilibrium in the healthcare market will enhance efficiency as well as outcomes.

Reduce Downward Healthcare Market Pressures

The current situation affecting the US healthcare market is far from desirable. Numerous pressures on the market hinder growth, progress, and innovation as well as efficiency and value. Among the most obvious pressures are those related to regulatory oversights, the increase in chronic disease burdens, aging populations, a lack of universal access, privacy and security issues, economic disparities, and health literacy issues. Each of these individually as well as all of them collectively serve to negatively affect the healthcare market in one way or another.

Certainly, addressing each of these issues is needed, and conversations about solutions for each is being pursued. However, these pressures do not exist in a vacuum. Instead, each of these are interrelated and interdependent, and any solution must address all of these collectively in order to facilitate progress and innovation within the healthcare market as a whole. We must adopt a broad, comprehensive, and unified vision to guide reforms in the right direction. Though short-term fluctuations in any given area may occur, long-term reductions in downward market pressures will ultimately result. This is needed for lasting, effective healthcare reforms.

Foster Patient Accountability

In the current healthcare system, patient adherence remains a serious issue. Adherence is classically defined as an individual's compliance to medical instructions over time. Commonly, adherence is associated primarily with medication compliance, but in actuality, adherence encompasses a much broader area. Adherence not only involves filling and taking medication prescriptions as ordered, but it also involves compliance with healthcare appointments, dietary instructions, exercise recommendations, therapy sessions, and more. Knowledge of patients' lack of compliance is often lacking. In addition, few repercussions exist other than the natural consequences of poor medical management. While consequences are evident from a health perspective, additional consequences pertaining to healthcare costs are also present.

The statistics on poor medical adherence are staggering. Among patients with chronic diseases, roughly half comply with medical recommendations over time. The effects of nonadherence in patients with asthma, diabetes, and hypertension alone results in substantial costs and negative outcomes. The figures are even worse for adherence to prevention recommendations—less than a third of patients comply. A quarter of patients never fill a prescription provided by a physician. And these statistics are simply those that have been reported by surveys and research studies. Actual nonadherence rates in all of these areas are likely worse.

A number of barriers to medical adherence exist. Complexities involving recommendations limit understanding and compliance, and polypharmacy as well as multiple providers can similarly make following recommendations more challenging. Poor health literacy, treatment side effects and adverse events, poor provider-patient communications, and costs of treatment represent other barriers. Each of these areas deserves attention in an effort to improve patient care.

Before adherence can be effectively addressed, better information regarding adherence among patients is needed. At the present time, the only means by which adherence is routinely monitored is through patient questions at the time of follow-up and/or testing of specific parameters in select diseases periodically. Effective adherence programs should offer a means to monitor patient compliance, and the use of information technologies to provide ongoing data to various healthcare stakeholders about adherence offers one solution. Improved patient care can result through use of programs that socially reward good adherence, and also that provide greater opportunities for removing adherence barriers.

Utilize Innovation to Reduce Healthcare Costs

Innovation has always been a cornerstone for medicine and healthcare. A great deal of health and pathophysiological processes are unknown. Therefore, a never-ending supply of complex health issues and dilemmas demand continuous efforts to find solutions. Thus, innovation is not only inherent to advancement of healthcare, but is an essential component.

While innovation can aid healthcare in several ways, reducing healthcare costs is perhaps one of the most pressing areas where innovation can be best utilized. Healthcare is plagued with many area of waste and inefficiencies where innovation could make significant impacts. For example, overtreatment and excessive utilization of resources could be streamlined and improved, and care coordination and execution could be enhanced to eliminate costs. In addition, administrative complexities and bureaucracies could be improved while fraud and abuse better identified. These should be the primary targets for innovations since these account for a sizable percentage of healthcare costs presently.

Numerous fields and markets within healthcare support innovative technologies. Governmental support for biomedical research has consistently supported these innovations, and likewise, numerous academic centers have done the same. In addition, private industries invest heavily in innovation and technologies. Such industries include pharmaceutical companies, medical device makers, surgical instrumentation companies, and biotechnology firms. Today, new sectors are also involved in healthcare innovations. Specifically, informatics and HIT organizations are seeking innovative ways to address major healthcare problems. This area in particular offers great promise for the future of healthcare, and the ikioo Health Monitoring and Management system can play a significant role toward these goals.

Summary Overview of Health Market Directions for the Twenty-First Century

In order to attain a more effective US healthcare system for the coming decades, this chapter has identified several areas and strategies we need to pursue. The current healthcare system is fraught with inefficiencies and waste, and it is burdened by excessive costs, regulatory constraints, and poorly aligned incentives. As a result, the healthcare market is nothing close to a free market system that allows competition and consumer demands to properly drive price and supply. The key to developing a better system thus lies in efforts to establish a free market environment so efficiency and value can again thrive.

Key efforts toward this end will involve a variety of strategies, including enhanced transparencies regarding costs, pricing, and cross-subsidizations as well as improved information sharing among all stakeholders. Likewise, economical health screenings of specific conditions in the population will need to be adopted as well as greater patient accountability regarding adherence. Other strategies will seek to create better market conditions through macro and micro efficiencies, better market equilibriums between supply and demand, and reductions in negative pressures on effective market activities. And incentives to promote innovation and the use of AI in HITs will be important.

Any comprehensive solution will require legislative actions and government involvement. This does not mean that continued regulation over reimbursement rates and pricing should continue; however, it will be necessary for legislative actions to guide market conditions. Such legislative actions will include efforts to align incentives toward value-based care, cost reductions, and waste elimination. Also, reevaluation of government subsidies should ensure such incentives are not only logical in pursuing value-based goals but similarly effective in their results. And legislation must address fair competition practices. While antitrust legislation must be maintained, other actions can promote greater competition, transparency, and information sharing, which would help better approximate a free market environment.

Clearly, a sweeping change in healthcare legislation will not be an end-all solution for the US healthcare system. Because of the changing nature of healthcare, ongoing and frequent analyses and reassessments must occur, and legislation must be changed according to these results. In addition, government actions alone will not resolve current issues. For example, providers must eliminate barriers to entry that currently hinder adequate supply to meet the growing consumer demand. However, by continually assessing system incentives to promote a free market environment, these actions by other stakeholders become increasingly likely. This is why government involvement is both needed and necessary to evoke effective change.

In these pursuits, AI and mobile HITs offer tremendous opportunities to realize key goals for healthcare reform. Potential advantages include better communications and collaborations among all healthcare stakeholders, better transparency and information sharing, enhanced provider decision-making capacities, and greater insights and knowledge based on data analytics. AI also has the ability to promote patient accountability and self-care while extending care environments well beyond the office and hospital settings. Through the use of AI and HITs, costs can be reduced in healthcare while efficiency, outcomes, and safety can be augmented.

The ikioo Health Monitoring and Management system reflects the use of such technologies as a means to pursue better healthcare systems and practices. By promoting an on-demand, on-the-go, and away-from-hospital care platform, healthcare services can be provided in real-time rather than piecemeal, and marked improvements in care efficiency can be attained. In addition, the ikioo system reestablishes a strong provider-patient relationship while allowing physicians to provide nuanced, personalized care based on unique individualized data. Many strategies will be needed to reform healthcare effectively, but the ikioo Health Monitoring and Management system does represent a key piece of this solution for the future. Through its use, physicians will be better equipped for healthcare in the twenty-first century.

About the Author

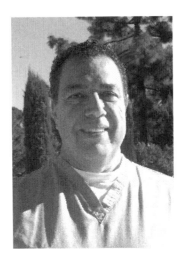

Ayman Salem, M. D. is a neurosurgeon and the founder of ikioo®
Technologies, Inc., in Burbank, California. His passion is to enhance
US and worldwide health care delivery via cutting edge artificial
intelligence algorithms. He is committed to building an open AI platform that would accommodate medicine as an art and as a profession.
His tireless work in fighting brain, spine and nerve disorders made
him realize that it is a shared fight. The more he listened and learned
from his patients, he came to realize that they care more about health
rather than disease. He felt that time has come for a total paradigm
shift in the way providers approach healthcare problems in the US
and worldwide.

Made in the USA
San Bernardino, CA
13 February 2017